AF845970

STRATEGIES TO LEVERAGE RESEARCH FUNDING

Guiding DOD's Peer Reviewed Medical Research Programs

Committee on Alternative Funding Strategies for DOD's Peer Reviewed Medical Research Programs

Medical Follow-Up Agency
and
Board on Health Sciences Policy

Michael McGeary and Kathi E. Hanna, Editors

INSTITUTE OF MEDICINE
OF THE NATIONAL ACADEMIES

THE NATIONAL ACADEMIES PRESS
Washington, D.C.
www.nap.edu

THE NATIONAL ACADEMIES PRESS 500 Fifth Street, NW Washington, DC 20001

NOTICE: The project that is the subject of this report was approved by the Governing Board of the National Research Council, whose members are drawn from the councils of the National Academy of Sciences, the National Academy of Engineering, and the Institute of Medicine. The members of the committee responsible for the report were chosen for their special competences and with regard for appropriate balance.

This study was supported by Contract No. W81XWH-04-C-0077 between the National Academy of Sciences and the U.S. Department of Defense. Any opinions, findings, conclusions, or recommendations expressed in this publication are those of the author(s) and do not necessarily reflect the view of the organizations or agencies that provided support for this project.

Library of Congress Cataloging-in-Publication Data

Strategies to leverage research funding : guiding DOD's peer reviewed medical research programs / Committee on Alternative Funding Strategies for DOD's Peer Reviewed Medical Research Programs, Medical Follow-Up Agency and Board on Health Sciences Policy ; Michael McGeary and Kathi E. Hanna, editors.
p. ; cm.
Includes bibliographical references.
ISBN 0-309-09277-9 (pbk.)
1. Medicine—Research—United States—Finance. 2. United States. Dept. of Defense.
[DNLM: 1. United States. Dept. of Defense. 2. Biomedical Research—economics—United States. 3. Research Support—methods—United States. W 20.5 S8986 2004] I. McGeary, Michael G. H. II. Hanna, Kathi E. III. Committee on Alternative Funding Strategies for DOD's Peer Reviewed Medical Research Programs.
R854.U5S754 2004
362.1′072′073—dc22

2004022342

Additional copies of this report are available from the National Academies Press, 500 Fifth Street, N.W., Lockbox 285, Washington, DC 20055; (800) 624-6242 or (202) 334-3313 (in the Washington metropolitan area); Internet, http://www.nap.edu.

For more information about the Institute of Medicine, visit the IOM home page at: **www.iom.edu.**

Printed in the United States of America.

The serpent has been a symbol of long life, healing, and knowledge among almost all cultures and religions since the beginning of recorded history. The serpent adopted as a logotype by the Institute of Medicine is a relief carving from ancient Greece, now held by the Staatliche Museen in Berlin.

"Knowing is not enough; we must apply.
Willing is not enough; we must do."
—Goethe

INSTITUTE OF MEDICINE
OF THE NATIONAL ACADEMIES

Adviser to the Nation to Improve Health

THE NATIONAL ACADEMIES

Advisers to the Nation on Science, Engineering, and Medicine

The **National Academy of Sciences** is a private, nonprofit, self-perpetuating society of distinguished scholars engaged in scientific and engineering research, dedicated to the furtherance of science and technology and to their use for the general welfare. Upon the authority of the charter granted to it by the Congress in 1863, the Academy has a mandate that requires it to advise the federal government on scientific and technical matters. Dr. Bruce M. Alberts is president of the National Academy of Sciences.

The **National Academy of Engineering** was established in 1964, under the charter of the National Academy of Sciences, as a parallel organization of outstanding engineers. It is autonomous in its administration and in the selection of its members, sharing with the National Academy of Sciences the responsibility for advising the federal government. The National Academy of Engineering also sponsors engineering programs aimed at meeting national needs, encourages education and research, and recognizes the superior achievements of engineers. Dr. Wm. A. Wulf is president of the National Academy of Engineering.

The **Institute of Medicine** was established in 1970 by the National Academy of Sciences to secure the services of eminent members of appropriate professions in the examination of policy matters pertaining to the health of the public. The Institute acts under the responsibility given to the National Academy of Sciences by its congressional charter to be an adviser to the federal government and, upon its own initiative, to identify issues of medical care, research, and education. Dr. Harvey V. Fineberg is president of the Institute of Medicine.

The **National Research Council** was organized by the National Academy of Sciences in 1916 to associate the broad community of science and technology with the Academy's purposes of furthering knowledge and advising the federal government. Functioning in accordance with general policies determined by the Academy, the Council has become the principal operating agency of both the National Academy of Sciences and the National Academy of Engineering in providing services to the government, the public, and the scientific and engineering communities. The Council is administered jointly by both Academies and the Institute of Medicine. Dr. Bruce M. Alberts and Dr. Wm. A. Wulf are chair and vice chair, respectively, of the National Research Council.

www.national-academies.org

COMMITTEE ON ALTERNATIVE FUNDING STRATGIES FOR DOD'S PEER REVIEWED MEDICAL RESEARCH PROGRAMS

Joseph S. Pagano, *Chair*, Lineberger Professor of Cancer Research and Director Emeritus, Lineberger Comprehensive Cancer Center, University of North Carolina School of Medicine
Samuel Broder, Executive Vice President, Celera Genomics, Rockville, Maryland (member until May 25, 2004)
Eric G. Campbell, Assistant Professor, Institute for Health Policy, Department of Medicine, Massachusetts General Hospital, Harvard Medical School
Thomas C. Caskey, President and Chief Executive Officer, Cogene Biotech Ventures, Ltd., Houston, Texas
Robert Cook-Deegan, Director, Center for Genome Ethics, Law, and Policy, Institute for Genome Sciences and Policy, Duke University
Maryann Feldman, Chair, Technical Innovation and Entrepreneurship and Professor of Business Economics, Rotman School of Management, University of Toronto
MaryAnn Guerra, Vice President, Research Operations, Translational Genomics Research Institute, Phoenix, Arizona
Musa Mayer, Consumer and Author, New York
Frank E. Samuel, Jr., Science and Technology Advisor to Governor of Ohio

Project Staff

Michael McGeary, Study Director, Medical Follow-Up Agency
Reine Y. Homawoo, Senior Program Assistant, Medical Follow-Up Agency
David Butler, Senior Program Officer, Board on Health Promotion and Disease Prevention (July 2004)
Jennifer Pinkerman, Research Associate, Medical Follow-Up Agency (through May 2004)
Susan McCutchen, Research Associate, Division of Behavioral and Social Sciences and Education (June 2004)
Kathi E. Hanna, Consultant
Sara Davidson Maddox, Editor

IOM Staff

Frederick (Rick) Erdtmann, Director, Medical Follow-Up Agency
Andrew Pope, Director, Board on Health Sciences Policy
Pamela Ramey-McCray, Administrative Assistant, Medical Follow-Up Agency
Andrea Cohen, Financial Associate

Reviewers

This report has been reviewed in draft form by individuals chosen for their diverse perspectives and technical expertise, in accordance with procedures approved by the NRC's Report Review Committee. The purpose of this independent review is to provide candid and critical comments that will assist the institution in making its published report as sound as possible and to ensure that the report meets institutional standards for objectivity, evidence, and responsiveness to the study charge. The review comments and draft manuscript remain confidential to protect the integrity of the deliberative process. We wish to thank the following individuals for their review of this report:

Irwin Feller
Emeritus Professor of Economics
Institute for Policy Research and Evaluation
Pennsylvania State University

Mauro Ferrari
Ohio State University
National Cancer Institute

Mark Frankel
Program Director
American Association for the Advancement of Science

Hedvig Hricak
Chair, Department of Radiology
Memorial Sloan-Kettering Cancer Center

Jerald Sadoff
Chief Executive Officer
Aeras Global TB Vaccine Foundation

Richard L. Sprott
Executive Director
Ellison Medical Foundation

Thomas P. Stossel
American Cancer Society Professor of Medicine
Harvard Medical School

Palmer W. Taylor
Sandra & Monroe Trout Professor of Pharmacology
Dean, School of Pharmacy & Pharmaceutical Sciences
University of California, San Diego

Although the reviewers listed above have provided many constructive comments and suggestions, they were not asked to endorse the conclusions or recommendations nor did they see the final draft of the report before its release. The review of this report was overseen by **Robert A. Frosch** and **Peter M. Howley**. Appointed by the National Research Council and Institute of Medicine, respectively, they were responsible for making certain that an independent examination of this report was carried out in accordance with institutional procedures and that all review comments were carefully considered. Responsibility for the final content of this report rests entirely with the authoring committee and the institution.

Preface

In 1992, in response to efforts of breast cancer survivors to direct more funding to understanding breast cancer and new and better ways to treat it, the U.S. Congress inserted a line-item in the fiscal year (FY) 1993 appropriation for the Department of Defense (DOD) that provided $210 million for peer-reviewed research on breast cancer. The U.S. Army Medical Research and Material Command implemented the congressional mandate by establishing the Breast Cancer Research Program (BCRP). Congress has not only continued to insert a line-item in the DOD budget each year for BCRP, it has added line-items for research on neurofibromatosis (FY 1996), prostate cancer (FY 1997), ovarian cancer (FY 1997), chronic myelogenous leukemia (FY 2002), tuberous sclerosis (FY 2002), and prion diseases (transmissible spongiform encephalopathies) (FY 2002). In addition, in FY 1999, Congress established a program of peer-reviewed research on military service-related topics, such as laser eye injury and trauma care.

Collectively, these mandated activities are known as the Department of Defense Congressionally Directed Medical Research Programs (CDMRP). In recent years, CDMRP appropriations have totaled more than $350 million and funded more than 700 new awards annually to investigators in university, non-profit research institutes, and in industrial, state government, and federal laboratories throughout the United States.

CDMRP is distinguished by its emphasis on innovation, especially in translational research, achieved primarily by supporting new ideas and bringing in new investigators. CDMRP uses a peer review system recommended by a 1993 Institute of Medicine (IOM) report that was modeled after the National Institutes of Health (NIH) system, but with a notable addition, the participation—not just representation—of patient advocates, then unprecedented and still unusual in government research programs. The peer review system is two-tiered, first reviewing research proposals for scientific quality, then reviewing them for programmatic relevance. Consumer advocates serve on both the first and the second-tier panels. CDMRP's performance has met with the approval of scientists, the satisfaction of legislators and their constituents, pride on the part of the program's administrators, and results.

In 1992, DOD was downsizing in response to the end of the Cold War, and it was relatively easy to find room in the DOD budget for a program meeting an urgent public need. Today, in the aftermath of the September 11, 2001, terrorist attack, DOD's budget situation is different. DOD's mission has expanded to fight wars in Afghanistan and Iraq and maintain the peace in other hot spots around the world, and the demands on the DOD budget have escalated. There is heavy downward pressure on the other activities of DOD, including CDMRP, which had a budget of more than $390 million as recently as FY 2002.

At the direction of Congress, DOD asked the Institute of Medicine to conduct a study exploring the possibility of attracting nonfederal funds to augment CDMRP's appropriated funds. The IOM appointed a committee to identify sources and means of nonfederal funding that could augment CDMRP's resources and strengthen it through creative partnering.

The Committee was well aware of the larger context for biomedical research support, in which tight budgets not only affect CDMRP but also the largest source of public funds, the National Institutes of Health. Importantly, the charge was not to evaluate CDMRP or recommend whether it should be maintained, curtailed, or phased out nor to consider other sources of federal co-funding, such as NIH. Rather the task given was to assess the potential for leveraging nonfederal resources to achieve the goals of CDMRP.

Members of the Committee sought to identify some innovative collaborative funding arrangements that CDMRP could use and that also could serve as models for other federal agencies and searched for imaginative solutions. For example, the Committee reviewed a variety of examples of innovative public-private cost sharing, partnerships, and other joint ventures in support of research and development (R&D), not only involving federal agencies, but also state and international agencies (examples are briefly described in Appendix A). A two-day workshop with presentations from representatives of nonfederal funding sources—including foundations, voluntary health agencies, universities, state research and economic development agencies, industry and venture capital—as well as of exemplary public-private research collaborations—was most informative and set the bases for models and sources that the Committee might realistically recommend (the workshop agenda is in Appendix C). Also, the Committee commissioned a paper reviewing economic studies of public-private collaboration in R&D and looked at the literature on the uses of cost-sharing and matching to augment federal research budgets (the paper is in Appendix D).

The report that follows assesses the extent of nonfederal sources of funding for research and details a variety of opportunities for leveraging nonfederal funding from the numerous sources examined. There are many examples in which the coordination of effort or the pooling of resources, or both, have leveraged research results that could not have been achieved otherwise. At the same time, the report is realistic about the extent to which these joint efforts are likely to generate a significant amount of additional resources for CDMRP.

The Committee would like to thank the many individuals and organizations that provided information and expert judgment, especially those who participated in the workshop on short notice. They and their organizational affiliations are listed in the agenda for the workshop (Appendix C). Several organizations submitted statements which were carefully considered by the committee—the Amyotrophic Lateral Sclerosis Association on April 27, 2004, during the public statement period of the workshop, and the National Coalition for Osteoporosis and Related Bone Diseases on May 20, 2004, by letter. Others who assisted were Greg Downing, National Cancer Institute; Neil Buckholtz and Susan Molchan, National Institute on Aging; James Schuttinga and Karen Pla, Office of the NIH Director; John Lowe and Kelly Robbins of the Henry M. Jackson Foundation for the Advancement of Military Medicine; Geoffrey Frisch of the Centers for Disease Control Foundation; and John Moore, CDC. The CDMRP staff was most helpful, including the director, Col. Kenneth Bertram, M.D., Ph.D., deputy director, Lt. Col. Calvin Carpenter, and several program directors, including Patricia Modrow, Ph.D., Leo Giambarresi, Ph.D., and Richard H. Kenyon, Ph.D.

I would like to thank the members of the Committee, who took on this assignment on short notice and attended three meetings and the workshop in a compressed time frame. The mix of expertise and experience was stimulating and well suited for the task. We learned from each other and came to know and regard well this significant biomedical research enterprise of the Department of Defense.

Finally, I would like to thank the study staff for the superb job they did at all levels despite the constraints imposed by a six-month deadline.

Joseph S. Pagano, M.D.
Chair

Contents

Figures, Tables, and Boxes

FIGURES

TABLES

BOXES

Abbreviations and Acronyms

AAFRC	American Association of Fundraising Counsel
ABC²	Accelerate Brain Cancer Cure
ABCC	administrative and bioinformatics coordinating center
ACCP	Alliance for Cervical Cancer Prevention
AD	Alzheimer's disease
ADA	American Diabetes Association
ADNI	Alzheimer's Disease Neuroimaging Initiative
AHA	American Heart Association
AICR	American Institute for Cancer Research
ALS	amyotrophic lateral sclerosis
AP4	Academic Public-Private Partnership Program
ARL	Army Research Laboratory
ARMF	Applied Research Matching Fund
ATP	Advanced Technology Program
AUTM	Association of University Technology Managers
BCRP	Breast Cancer Research Program
BIO	Biotechnology Industry Organization
BRCA1	breast cancer 1 gene
Bt	*Bacillus thuringiensis*
CAD	Canadian dollar
CAL-(IT)²	California Institute for Telecommunications and Information Technology

CBCRP	California Breast Cancer Research Program
CDC	Centers for Disease Control and Prevention
CDMRP	Congressionally Directed Medical Research Programs
CF	cystic fibrosis
CFF	Cystic Fibrosis Foundation
CFFT	Cystic Fibrosis Foundation Therapeutics, Inc.
CIA	Central Intelligence Agency
CIHR	Canadian Institutes of Health Research
CITRIS	Center for Information Technology Research in the Interest of Society
CMLRP	Chronic Myelogenous Leukemia Research Program
CNSI	California Nanosystems Institute
CRADA	Cooperative Research and Development Agreement
CSI	Congressional Special Interest
CSO	Common Scientific Outline
DARPA	Defense Advanced Research Projects Agency
DCA	Defense Cooperation Account
DFID	Department for International Development
DHHS	Department of Health and Human Services
DNA	deoxyribonucleic acid
DOD	Department of Defense
DOE	Department of Energy
DTI	Department of Trade and Industry
DUS&T	Dual Use Science and Technology (DUS&T) Program
EMBRAPA	Brazilian Agricultural Research Corporation (Empresa Brasileira de Pesquisa Agropecuária)
EPA	Environmental Protection Agency
ERC	Engineering Research Center
FDA	Food and Drug Administration
FNIH	Foundation for the National Institutes of Health
FY	fiscal year
GC	Genome Canada
GICUR	Government/Industry Co-sponsorship of University Research Program
GUIRR	Government-University-Industry Research Roundtable
HEFCE	Higher Education Funding Council of England
HEI	Health Effects Institute
HER2	Human Epidermal Growth Factor Receptor 2

HHMI	Howard Hughes Medical Institute
HIPAA	Health Insurance Portability and Accountability Act
HTP	Human Transcriptome Project
IAVI	International AIDS Vaccine Initiative
ICR	Islet Cell Resource Center
IDEA	Innovative Developmental and Exploratory Awards
IOM	Institute of Medicine
IP	intellectual property
ISS	International Space Station
ITN	Immune Tolerance Network
I/UCRC	Industry/University Cooperative Research Centers Program
IUCRP	Industry-University Cooperative Research Program
JDRF	Juvenile Diabetes Research Foundation International
JIF	Joint Infrastructure Fund
KTEC	Kansas Technology Enterprise Corporation
LLNL	Lawrence Livermore National Laboratory
MARCO	Microelectronics Advanced Research Corporation
MDA	Muscular Dystrophy Association
MDCRC	Muscular Dystrophy Cooperative Research Center Program
MIM	Multilateral Initiative on Malaria
MMV	Medicines for Malaria Venture
MRSEC	Materials Research Science and Engineering Centers Program
MSC	Mouse Sequencing Consortium
MTA-CRADA	material transfer agreement CRADA
NASA	National Aeronautics and Space Administration
NBCC	National Breast Cancer Coalition
NCBC	North Carolina Biotechnology Center
NCI	National Cancer Institute
NCRA	National Cooperative Research Act
NCRR	National Center for Research Resources
NEI	National Eye Institute
NF	neurofibromatosis
NFRP	Neurofibromatosis Research Program
NGA	National Governors Association
NGO	nongovernmental organization
NHGRI	National Human Genome Research Institute
NHLBI	National Heart, Lung, and Blood Institute

NIA	National Institute on Aging
NIAID	National Institute of Allergy and Infectious Diseases
NIAMS	National Institute of Arthritis and Musculoskeletal and Skin Diseases
NICHD	National Institute of Child Health and Human Development
NCRR	National Center for Research Resources
NIDCR	National Institute of Dental and Craniofacial Research
NIDDK	National Institute of Diabetes and Digestive and Kidney Diseases
NIEHS	National Institute of Environmental Health Sciences
NIH	National Institutes of Health
NIMH	National Institute of Mental Health
NINDS	National Institute of Neurological Disorders and Stroke
NINR	National Institute of Nursing Research
NIST	National Institute of Standards and Technology
NSB	National Science Board
NSEC	Nanoscale Science and Engineering Centers Program
NSF	National Science Foundation
NVCA	National Venture Capital Association
OAI	Osteoarthritis Initiative
OCRP	Ovarian Cancer Research Program
OIG	Office of Inspector General
OIT	Ontario Innovation Trust
OMB	Office of Management and Budget
ORDCF	Ontario Research and Development Challenge Fund
ORMH	Office of Research on Minority Health
ORWH	Office of Research on Women's Health
OST	Office of Science and Technology
PCRP	Prostate Cancer Research Program
PFI	Partnerships for Innovation
PhRMA	Pharmaceutical Research and Manufacturers of America
PPP	public-private partnership
PRMRP	Peer Reviewed Medical Research Program
QB3	California Institute for Bioengineering, Biotechnology, and Quantitative Biomedical Research
R!A	Research!America
R&D	research and development
RAD	Research Area Directorate
RFA	Request for Applications

RFP	Request for Proposals
RJV	research joint venture
SARS	Severe Acute Respiratory Syndrome
SBIR	Small Business Innovation Research Program
SEMATECH	Semiconductor Manufacturing Technology Consortium
SGC	Structural Genomics Consortium
SPD	Space Partnership Development
SPORE	Specialized Programs of Research Excellence
SRIF	Science Research Investment Fund
SSTI	State Science and Technology Institute
STAR	Strategic Technology and Research Fund
STC	Science and Technology Center
STTR	Small Business Technology Transfer Program
T1DGC	International Type 1 Diabetes Genetics Consortium
TATRC	Telemedicine and Advanced Technology Research Center
TB	tuberculosis
TCRF	Technology Commercialization Research Fund
TDN	Therapeutic Development Network
TEDDY	Triggers and Environmental Determinants of Diabetes in Youth
TGEN	Translational Genomics Research Institute
TIA	Technology Investment Agreement
TMM	Technologies for Metabolic Monitoring
TOBI	tobramycin solution for inhalation
TSCRP	Tuberous Sclerosis Complex Research Program
UC	University of California
UK	United Kingdom
U.S.	United States
USAMRDC	U.S. Army Medical Research and Development Command
USAMRMC	U.S. Army Medical Research and Materiel Command
USDA	U.S. Department of Agriculture
VA	Department of Veterans Affairs
VHAs	voluntary health agencies
WHO	World Health Organization

Executive Summary

The Department of Defense's (DOD's) Congressionally Directed Medical Research Programs (CDMRP) originated in 1992 in response to a congressional mandate to create and manage a research effort aimed at ending breast cancer. It has expanded to include major research support efforts addressing prostate cancer, ovarian cancer, and neurofibromatosis, and smaller scale and short-term initiatives on other health problems. CDMRP is a program administered by the U.S. Army that supports research by scientists in universities, industrial laboratories, federal and state government agencies, and other research institutions. The program focuses on basic and clinical research and training and has developed a reputation for consumer participation in priority setting and peer review, innovative award mechanisms, and support of cutting-edge research. Unlike most federal health research support mechanisms, CDMRP is appropriated on a year-to-year basis with program-specific funding levels.

Recently, Congress became concerned about funding increases for CDMRP, because of competing demands on the military budget, especially the wars in Iraq and Afghanistan. In 2004, at congressional request, DOD asked the Institute of Medicine (IOM) to report on the possibilities of augmenting program funding from nonfederal sources. IOM was asked to form a committee to identify mechanisms that could be used to leverage such funding, assess the impacts of alternative nonfederal sources and mechanisms of funding on CDMRP, and identify any legal or regulatory barriers to leveraging nonfederal funding. The Committee on Alternative Funding Strategies for DOD's Peer Reviewed Biomedical Research Programs was not asked to evaluate CDMRP; recommend whether it should be continued, restructured, or phased out; or look at the potential for co-funding research with other federal programs.

The report focuses on nonfederal funding sources and mechanisms and their potential effects on the program if adopted. The committee identified many potential nonfederal sources but concluded that the prospects for augmenting CDMRP funding from these sources are modest, at best, especially regarding "new" funds that would not otherwise be devoted to biomedical research. Voluntary collaborations can, however, leverage research results that cannot be achieved by individual funders working separately, for example, through the creation of synergies, critical mass, economies of scale, and other ways that make the whole greater than the sum of its parts.

The committee found numerous examples of federal agencies leveraging nonfederal funds. One common approach is to require cost sharing or matching by grantees; another is to encourage voluntary public-private collaborations between government and other donors or between university grantees and industry. However, substantial cost sharing or matching is costly for grantees to secure and document and for the granting agency to oversee, while successful public-private funding collaborations depend on an alignment of interests among the contributing parties to carry out a particular project or program, which most commonly occurs with clinical research or research directed at the development of products (e.g., diagnostics, drugs, vaccines, devices).

CDMRP has the authority to require cost sharing by grant recipients (which it exercises by requiring awardee institutions to provide the facilities and equipment for conducting research projects and the faculty for training programs), but the program lacks the authority to accept private funds and a foundation would need to be established to solicit private funds for collaborative projects. The committee developed recommendations for CDMRP to facilitate federal funding that emphasize voluntary collaborations in funding research and that focus on providing CDMRP with the authority to engage in jointly funded projects and programs while ensuring that the best features of the current program are not undermined.

POTENTIAL SOURCES OF NONFEDERAL FUNDS

Sources of potential additional funding for medical research supported by DOD include for-profit companies, venture capital firms, foundations and other philanthropies, and state governments. Because CDMRP already collaborates and co-funds projects with other federal agencies, most notably the National Institutes of Health (NIH), the committee was asked to focus on nonfederal sources.

Approximately 10 percent of pharmaceutical industry expenditures on research and development (R&D) goes to basic research. Thus, industry spends a great deal of money on biomedical research, but little on the types of activities that the majority of CDMRP funding currently supports. First, industry is most interested in short-term research and development projects with commercial promise, such as the development of diagnostics, therapeutics, and devices and the creation of research tools and databases. Efforts to increase industry support of CDMRP programs could shift priorities toward such activities. Second, for-profit co-funding of awards to university scientists could introduce a number of issues and potential risks, including conflicts of interest for faculty who could benefit financially from their university research; increased secrecy and other restrictions on the dissemination of industrial research results; reduced faculty time commitments to the activities of the university; and the use of students in conducting privately funded research. Third, there is no avenue currently by which industry can contribute funding directly to CDMRP, although this problem could be remedied (see below).

Venture capital is invested in late-stage R&D, with the expectation of commercial products. Representatives of these sectors at the committee's workshop said that they would not be likely to give CDMRP a blank check by transferring funds to it directly and that they would expect to play a significant role in determining where their research dollars were spent. At the same time, they indicated strong interest in collaborating when mutual interests are identified.

It is a common strategy of philanthropies, state governments, and universities to leverage federal funds to achieve their goals. However, foundations and public charities, such as the American Cancer Society, have limited resources compared with the federal government, and they focus on funding activities that are not well supported by the federal government, such as public health, or on activities that leverage federal funding, such as providing grants for exploratory research and new investigators. Some foundations collaborate with federal agencies on projects of mutual interest and even give funds to agencies to expand programs, which would be beneficial, but the amounts of money are modest relative to the appropriations for CDMRP.

Most states have economic development programs that are interested in funding medical research and biotechnology, often using dollars that are new and that, until recently, would not have been spent on medical research. But states, like industry, are generally most interested in funding research that has immediate commercial application, because the ultimate goal of the research is to build the state's biotechnology industry and thus increase the number of jobs. Moreover, a principal thrust of most state economic development funds is to leverage multiple federal dollars for each state dollar, not the other way around. In addition, states must balance health research against other needs such as improved transit and the funding of manufacturing plants. In general, state research funds would be most available for biotechnology development and not innovative exploratory health research. Finally, strategies contingent on the availability of state funding would tend to direct federal funds to states that wish to mount research programs to parallel those of CDMRP and that already have the means to do so.

In general, nonfederal funding leveraged by CDMRP would not necessarily be "new" money that expands the overall amount of support for biomedical research. In most cases, the nonfederal funds would be redirected from other areas of biomedical research. For example, one effect of a cost-sharing requirement in CDMRP programs might be that charitable organizations will be called on to provide matching funds that they would have spent themselves on the same areas of research. Although the total amount spent on the CDMRP program would be increased, the overall amount of funding for biomedical research would not change. The principal difference would be the additional administrative effort required to account for funding streams and to secure agreement on co-funding arrangements.

In conclusion, there are many potential sources of nonfederal funding for CDMRP, although the amounts of additional funding they could contribute are likely to be limited because their priorities differ from CDMRP's research agenda. Nonfederal funders are least likely to fund exploratory research on new ideas or to support new investigators, which constitute the majority of CDMRP support. Nonfederal donors are most likely to be interested in collaborating on applied research and development work on potential products with near-term commercial payoffs—e.g., diagnostics, therapeutics, and devices. While collaborations might not leverage much funding, they can leverage research results by creating synergies or otherwise enabling research that cannot be done by individual funders, and CDMRP should take advantage of opportunities to achieve this kind of leverage.

MECHANISMS FOR SECURING OTHER FUNDING

Federal agencies that support R&D use a variety of mechanisms to leverage other funding. Broadly considered, these mechanisms fall into two groups. One set of mechanisms relies on requirements that awardees pay a portion of the costs of the project from nonfederal sources, called cost sharing or matching. The other set of mechanisms consists of voluntary collaborations between federal agencies and nonfederal donors in supporting research of mutual interest.

Cost-sharing or matching requirements are commonly used by agencies in development projects for which industry involvement is desired and from which industry stands to gain. Cost sharing is not usually required for programs that support basic research conducted by individual investigators or small research teams. CDMRP requires a small amount of cost sharing by expecting grantees to provide the facilities and equipment needed in the proposed research or, in the case of training grants, by paying for the mentoring and other nonstipend costs. Currently, CDMRP does not document the monetary value or extent of this cost sharing.

Matching fund requirements appear at first glance to be a good way to leverage funds but, for several reasons, they may not in fact increase the total amount of research. Indeed, they may add administrative costs and accounting complexity without funding additional research. First, matching funds may be diverted from other research projects. Second, they are not free. The principal investigators and institutional research administrators must spend additional time lining up matching fund donors, planning the project, and preparing a more complex application. The time and effort that researchers and administrators spend searching for funding is time not spent conducting research and augmenting knowledge. In addition, some highly promising research may not be funded because of a lack of matching funds, and funding may be redistributed from new investigators to better known investigators who could attract other funding, wealthier institutions with greater means to provide the matching funds, or states with research programs able to match CDMRP funding. Finally, both the awardee institution and CDMRP would have to expand their staffs to account for and audit the matching funds to ensure that they are legitimate and not counted as matching on another federal grant.

Expectations that the program should leverage substantial funds through matching requirements would be likely to shift program priorities from basic research toward applied research and development, particularly if the additional funding came from industry, which is more interested in supporting the later stages of the R&D process. Industry and states have funded fairly basic research activities in some cases, however, such as biomarker development and stem cell research centers.

If well planned, voluntary collaborations between CDMRP and other organizations and agencies in funding research could, however, be mutually beneficial in terms of enlarging the base of research leading to better health outcomes, achieving a critical mass of resources needed for progress in a research area, and/or promoting synergy among different sponsors with complementary knowledge, skills, techniques, and other resources. The funding arrangements involved in voluntary collaborations may include pooling funds for grants, but they also may include arrangements in which funding does not change hands, such as agreements to fund grants separately or to fund different but complementary parts of a project or for nonfederal donors to provide supplements to federal grantees.

Some federal agencies, such as NIH and the Centers for Disease Control and Prevention (CDC), have the authority to accept gifts for specified purposes and have foundations that can solicit private funds for their programs. If Congress wishes CDMRP to draw on foundations and private donors, it needs to create the authority to receive gifts to support research administered by CDMRP or in collaboration with CDMRP (see below).

ASSESSMENT OF ALTERNATIVE FUNDING SOURCES AND MECHANISMS FOR CDMRP

Despite initial skepticism in the scientific community about its location in DOD and the participation of consumers in peer review and priority setting,

CDMRP has shown that it has been an efficiently managed and scientifically productive effort and that it is a valuable component of the nation's health research enterprise. Distinctive program features include its rigorous peer review of proposals for scientific merit and program relevance by outside reviewers that includes consumers; its inclusive priority setting process; its emphasis on exploratory high-risk/high-gain basic, translational, and clinical research projects and on research capacity building; and its holding of periodic national meetings to share results among the investigators and with the program's constituencies.

Great care should be taken to ensure that changes in the program intended to leverage funding do not damage the features of the program that have made it efficient, driven by scientific priorities, and scientifically productive.

Currently, CDMRP has a relatively low administrative overhead of approximately 6 percent overall. Although increased cost-sharing requirements would impose costs chiefly on applicants and awardees, it also would require increased DOD staffing to ensure that those requirements are met. In addition, increased emphasis on raising outside funds for CDMRP programs would require additional staff to arrange and maintain relationships with the other funders. Likewise, establishing a foundation to plan collaborative programs and solicit funding from nonfederal sources would add to overhead costs.

CDMRP has used the two-tier review system recommended by the 1993 Institute of Medicine report to ensure that scientific quality and program relevance are the main determinants of the awards. Increased cost sharing would need to be carefully designed to ensure that the peer review system is not distorted, for example, by discouraging proposals from investigators representing institutions with little access to cost-sharing resources or by inciting a bidding war among applicants.

If CDMRP accepts funds from nonfederal sources—for example, donations from pharmaceutical or biotechnology companies to expand the pool of grants for a particular program of mutual interest—those funds should be distributed through the existing two-step peer review process to applicants who present the best proposals in terms of technical excellence and program relevance.

Currently, most funds appropriated to CDMRP support basic research, including a substantial number of exploratory grants. The program also supports new investigators and research programs in minority institutions. In addition, CDMRP funds research on the causes and prevention of the diseases these programs address. All of these are activities that industry is less likely to co-fund in favor of activities that support commercial development. Although foundations and disease charities do fund exploratory and basic research programs, and should be encouraged to engage in collaborations, their resources are relatively small when compared with those of industry or the federal government. The easiest way to attract nonfederal funding would be to change program priorities to emphasize the development and testing of drugs and vaccines and other efforts to develop commercial products; however, the advisability of such a shift is questionable given the amount of funding that industry and other federal agencies already devote to such activities and in light of the need for additional basic—especially exploratory—research in understanding the diseases that CDMRP addresses. Such a shift likely would increase the concentration of work in areas that already enjoy ample funding at the expense of support of new ideas and new investigators, CDMRP's signature area of strength.

As noted earlier, the risks of collaboration with for-profit firms include the imposition of secrecy on the scientific process, delays and bias in the reporting of research results, the shifting of research priorities toward near-term development rather than long-term research, and possibility of financial conflicts of interest for both research institutions and individual researchers. CDMRP would need to be aware of these risks, develop guidelines for industry collaborations, and be prepared to manage any conflicts.

CHANGES IN FEDERAL LAWS AND REGULATIONS REQUIRED BY ALTERNATIVE FUNDING SOURCES AND MECHANISMS

One mechanism for securing nonfederal funding for CDMRP to enlarge one or all of its grant programs would be through accepting voluntary contributions from foundations, companies, state governments, and other funders of medical research. As a model, the Secretary of Health and Human Services has statutory authority to accept conditional gifts for study, investigation, or research and other purposes, which has been delegated to the NIH director and the institute directors. CDC may also accept conditional gifts. Currently, according to the law which authorizes general gift funds, the recipient of contributions to the Army or DOD cannot be specified except for DOD hospitals, schools, and other health, education, and welfare activities. Other donations must be unconditional and appropriated by Congress before they can be used.

In order for CDMRP to accept nonfederal funds in support of a project or program, DOD would need statutory authorization to accept contributions from nonfederal donors for a specific purpose, for example, to fund research grants for a particular purpose. Based on NIH and CDC experience, however, the amounts of nonfederal funding would be very small compared with federal funding.

A related mechanism would be the establishment of a nonprofit foundation to solicit funds for CDMRP programs, because even if CDMRP were authorized to accept contributions, federal employees may not actively seek them to augment appropriated funds. To deal with this, some agencies, such as NIH and CDC, have foundations with staffs that seek donors for agency programs. For this to occur, Congress would need to charter a foundation similar to the ones it chartered for NIH and CDC or, possibly, expand the authority of the Henry M. Jackson Foundation for the Advancement of Military Medicine beyond its mission of supporting intramural research.

Grants and cooperative agreements for extramural research are subject to a number of conditions that may deter some commercial firms from doing business with the federal government. The Defense Advanced Research Projects Agency and the military departments (including the Army) have special authority to enter into transactions other than contracts, grants, and cooperative agreements. Such "other transactions" are exempt from the usual controls and oversight mechanisms set forth in acquisition statutes and the Federal Acquisition Regulation and from laws applying only to contracts, grants, and cooperative agreements. Under this authority, DOD has established an assistance instrument called the Technology Investment Agreement (TIA) in which DOD partners with a company or consortium of companies which contributes half or more of the costs of the project. TIAs were created to increase the participation in defense R&D of for-profit firms that are reluctant to comply with traditional instruments whose requirements or procedures are considered too burdensome, intrusive, or costly. In a TIA, for example, DOD may negotiate less restrictive intellectual property rights than are required by the Bayh-Dole Act.

TIAs are most appropriate when CDMRP is trying to stimulate product or technology development with enough commercial promise that a firm or firms would be willing to pay half the costs. The Secretary of the Army would need to delegate the authorities to award and administer TIAs to CDMRP.

RECOMMENDATIONS

The committee determined that it would be possible to leverage nonfederal funds, but only to a limited extent for certain types of research that are not the main focus of the CDMRP program. This includes later-stage research with potential near-term applications that are likely to be commercially viable, a type of research that already is supported by major medical research funders. The possibility of obtaining co-funding from industry, the largest nonfederal funder by far, is least likely for early-stage exploratory research, which has been CDMRP's most important contribution. It would be desirable for CDMRP to pursue the leveraging of outside funds for later-stage research, but only to the extent it does not unduly shift the program's priorities as set by its advisory panels. Leveraging would be facilitated if Congress granted the authority and means for CDMRP to solicit and use outside funds for extramural awards. Finally, the risks inherent in public-private collaborations must be addressed and managed.

The findings and recommendations that follow are not likely to result in a significant influx of new outside funding into CDMRP, primarily because of the program's high-risk focus on innovation, a focus that is properly the function of government, not the private sector.

Recommendation 1: Facilitate Collaboration When Appropriate

Findings. The majority of biomedical research funding comes from industry and is not readily accessible to a program such as CDMRP. Experience with cost sharing in other federal basic research programs shows that requiring recipients to provide significant percentages of the cost of projects to augment federal funds imposes additional expenses on both the recipient and the funder. This requirement also can have unintended—and often unwanted—consequences (such as discouraging the submission of outstanding proposals from researchers at institutions with limited means), and may not substantially increase the total amount of funding in an area of research (or may redirect it from other important uses). Cost sharing is most appropriate when the co-funder receives a tangible benefit, and this is much more likely to happen in later-stage research or infrastructure projects than in basic and exploratory research. Yet CDMRP's greatest strength has been its support of new ideas and new investigators, where cost sharing beyond the provision of facilities and equipment is least justified.

The experience of federal R&D funding agencies with voluntary public-private collaborations generally has been positive, although collaborations must be individually negotiated, which can add significant costs to a project and increase the time it takes for the research to begin. Appendix A includes a number of examples in which foundations, companies, and state governments have partnered with federal agencies in a research project or program.

Recommendation 1. CDMRP should facilitate collaborative arrangements for funding research when collaboration would be beneficial and appropriate—for example, when it would achieve greater results through synergy or economies of scale or critical mass—but CDMRP should not expect such arrangements to augment significantly overall program funding.

Opportunities for collaboration with other sponsors of biomedical R&D should be encouraged, not to stretch program funds, but rather to achieve program goals that could not be met otherwise. For example, increased funding might allow attainment of a critical mass in an area that no single funder could achieve by itself, development of a shared infrastructure, or the creation of a synergistic effect through the interactions of the different collaborators.

CDMRP should experiment with award mechanisms that facilitate collaborative R&D arrangements among academic institutions, industry, philanthropies, state governments, and/or other supporters of research, as has been done in the Breast Cancer Research Program with Collaborative-Clinical Translational Research Awards and Biotechnology Clinical Partnerships. In addition, CDMRP should, through its inclusive planning process, develop programs that outside funders would be willing to help fund (see Recommendation 2, below, for a private foundation to be set up to solicit and transfer such funds). An alternative would be for CDMRP to approach nonfederal funders to explore the possibility that they might fund projects that receive high scores but that cannot be funded by CDMRP. This reliance on the CDMRP application and review process would save the nonfederal funders administrative costs.

Recommendation 2: Provide DOD with Gift Authority

Findings. Some federal agencies, such as NIH and CDC, have authority to accept gifts for specified purposes and have foundations that can solicit private funds for their programs. Under current law and regulations, however, the Army is only allowed to accept private donations in its Army General Gift Fund for certain purposes (e.g., to benefit a school, hospital, library, museum, cemetery, or similar Army institution or organization), which do not include augmenting the funding of an extramural grant program such as CDMRP. Unlike some of these other federal research agencies, neither CDMRP nor its parent organization, the U.S. Army Medical Research and Materiel Command (USAMRMC), has the authority to receive outside funds to augment its budget for extramural awards. Even if it had such authority, it could not be used actively, as it is not legal for federal employees to seek funds from private sources.

The Henry M. Jackson Foundation for the Advancement of Military Medicine was established to be the recipient of funding for medical research and education projects from other federal and nonfederal sources, but only on behalf of the faculty of the Uniformed Services University of the Health Sciences, researchers at Walter Reed Army Institute of Research, and other intramural DOD researchers. The Jackson Foundation does not fund extramural research. Nonfederal funders also may contribute funds to the Defense Cooperation Account (DCA), but Congress must appropriate these funds and authorize their use for a specific purpose, and donors are asked not to designate the intended use of their contributions to DCA. If Congress wishes CDMRP to draw on foundations and private donors, it needs to create the authority to receive gifts to support research administered by CDMRP or in collaboration with CDMRP.

Recommendation 2. Congress should provide CDMRP with authority to:

a. receive gifts and donations from individuals, companies, foundations, and other organizations for the support of research grants and contracts awarded by CDMRP, and
b. charter a nonprofit foundation with authority to solicit and transfer nonfederal funds for the support of research grants and contracts awarded by CDMRP.

Gift authority might be granted to the Secretary of Defense, the Service Secretaries, or the Commander of USAMRMC, as long as it is delegated to the CDMRP program. A nonprofit foundation with the mission of assisting CDMRP or USAMRMC could be modeled after the Foundation for the National Institutes of Health or the CDC Foundation. Alternatively, the mission of the Henry M. Jackson Foundation could be expanded to include fundraising for CDMRP or USAMRMC extramural research programs. Based on the experience of similar foundations for other agencies, however, expectations of substantial donations to such a foundation should be modest. Congress also would have to provide for the additional costs of establishing and maintaining the foundation.

Recommendation 3: Limit Cost-Sharing/Matching Requirements

Findings. Cost sharing and matching requirements do not always advance research goals. Usually, cost-shared funds do not expand the total funding provided for research. Rather, they involve the rechanneling of existing funding streams. In addition, cost-sharing requirements can impose additional administrative costs on both recipients and funders. However, cost sharing makes sense where the extra costs are more than offset by additional benefits resulting from the partnership, such as when research results have foreseeable commercial applications.

Recommendation 3. CDMRP should not impose cost-sharing or matching fund requirements beyond those currently required, except when a tangible benefit to the award recipient is anticipated beyond the immediate term or scope of CDMRP-supported activity (for example, funding of instruments and facilities).

Care should be taken to see that cost sharing does not divert funds from other desirable activities, such as other research projects that would have been funded by those dollars. CDMRP should not let expectations of increased nonfederal funding shift the program's scientific priorities away from its focus on innovative exploratory research, research into disease prevention and causation, and epidemiological studies.

Recommendation 4: Issue Guidelines for Collaboration

Findings. Research on university-industry and government-industry partnerships and similar collaborations has identified a number of potential benefits and costs. The benefits generally take the form of induced private investment in developing research results into commercial goods and services, but these benefits do not necessarily require co-funding or formal matching requirements. The costs can include the imposition of secrecy on the scientific process, the occurrence of delays and bias in the reporting of research results, the shifting of research priorities toward near-term development rather than long-term research, and the possibility of financial conflicts of interest for both research institutions and individual researchers.

Recommendation 4. DOD should issue guidelines for collaboration with the private sector, paying special attention to the potential impact of research collaborations with nonfederal funders on (a) program costs; (b) the integrity of the peer review process; (c) program priorities;

(d) perceived and actual conflicts of interest; (e) openness in scientific communication, and (f) other issues that may arise in federal-private co-funding arrangements.

Other research funding agencies such as NIH and CDC have issued guidelines, which could serve as models for DOD guidelines. They focus on such issues as potential conflicts of interest that must be identified and addressed; intellectual property rights; the timely publication of research results; and the maintenance of academic freedom, and they contain suggestions of ways to avoid or manage them.

1

Introduction

DOD'S CONGRESSIONALLY DIRECTED MEDICAL RESEARCH PROGRAMS

The U.S. Army, on behalf of the Department of Defense (DOD), administers a set of biomedical research programs that support basic, translational, and clinical research projects; research training; and research infrastructure for specific diseases identified by Congress. The programs consist of awards that are made to extramural investigators and that are selected through a two-stage external peer review process that includes scientists, clinicians, and consumer advocates. In recent years, Congress has earmarked approximately $350 million per year in total for these programs, called collectively the Congressionally Directed Medical Research Programs (CDMRP).

Origin of the Program

CDMRP was initiated in 1992 in response to several forces. One was the emergence of women's health as an urgent public policy issue. In July 1991, for example, the *New England Journal of Medicine* published several studies showing that there was sex bias in the management of coronary heart disease. In addition, the National Institutes of Health (NIH) had recently launched a women's health initiative and was requiring the inclusion of women in clinical trials.

At the same time, concern about breast cancer specifically was being mobilized by a new grassroots organization, the National Breast Cancer Coalition

(NBCC), which was created in May 1991 (Casamayou, 2001). In October 1991, NBCC's efforts generated 600,000 letters to Congress and the White House that asked for increased spending on breast cancer research, and in February 1992, NBCC held research hearings during which leading breast cancer scientists identified research needs. On the basis of this meeting, NBCC began to campaign for "$300 million more" for cancer research and emphasized the need to fund research in ways that were different from those employed by traditional federal medical research agencies (Visco, 2004).

Lobbying by breast cancer groups had previously resulted in congressionally mandated funding increases for breast cancer research at DOD and the National Cancer Institute (NCI) in the fiscal year (FY) 1992 federal budget. The DOD budget earmarked $25 million for research on the screening and diagnosis of breast cancer among military medical beneficiaries and their dependents. Congress also directed NCI to increase its efforts in breast cancer research, as well as prostate and ovarian cancer research, by $100 million in FY 1992. However, the Budget Enforcement Act of 1990 imposed a strict cap on budget increases in domestic discretionary programs, and an increase of only $30 million was provided to NCI in FY 1992. Even with this increase, cuts in existing cancer research programs were necessary to accommodate the new mandates from Congress. This was the first time that cuts in ongoing cancer research programs were required to provide increases for new cancer research initiatives.

In addition, although this budget increase raised breast cancer research spending at NCI to $133 million in FY 1992, this was still substantially less than the $300 million urged by NBCC. As a result, many members of the cancer research and advocacy communities, spearheaded by NBCC, worked with Congress to identify a source of new funds for breast cancer research that would not further reduce the funding for existing cancer research programs.

One attractive source of funding at that time was DOD, which had approximately $29 billion in unobligated funds from prior years for the development of weapons systems planned before collapse of the Soviet Union in 1991.[1] Those funds were put off limits by the Budget Enforcement Act of 1990, which established "firewalls" between the budgets for defense, foreign affairs, and domestic programs and imposed strict caps on funding increases in each of the three categories. A number of attempts were made to breach the firewalls by transferring defense funding to domestic programs, including two attempts in September 1992 that would have increased funding for breast cancer research specifically, but they all failed.[2] Ultimately, Senator Tom Harkin put forward an amendment

---

[1]Congressional Budget Office estimate quoted by Senator Arlen Specter during debate on the Harkin transfer amendment in September 1992 (*Congressional Record*, September 16, 1992, p. S13594).

[2]Senator Harkin proposed a amendment to the Senate Labor-HHS-Education Appropriations bill for FY 1993 that would have taken $4.1 billion from the defense budget to augment programs in the

to the FY 1993 defense budget to increase funding for breast cancer research *within* DOD (rather than at NIH) by $185 million, to bring the total breast cancer research program within DOD to $210 million (Watson, 1992). As a transfer within DOD's research and development (R&D) budget, the amendment did not violate the budget agreement's firewalls. The funds were to be taken from the Strategic Defense Initiative and thus would be above and beyond the battlefield medicine-oriented core program of the U.S. Army Medical Research and Materiel Command (USAMRMC),[3] which was funded at $410 million in the Senate bill. The "Harkin Amendment for Breast Cancer" which passed in the Senate by a vote of 89 to 4, also stipulated that all projects funded by the resulting Breast Cancer Research Program (BCRP) would have to undergo peer review (Mervis, 1993).

During the debate on the amendment, Senator Harkin indicated his intent to have these funds made available to the cancer research community by the Army in collaboration with NCI. (NCI itself was slated to receive $220 million for breast cancer research in the Senate version of the FY 1993 appropriation act for NIH).[4]

Initial Establishment of the Program

Discussions between USAMRMC and NIH about participating in the setting of research priorities and the review of proposals broke down (*Science*, 1992; *Washington Fax*, 1992), and the USAMRMC contracted with the Institute of Medicine (IOM) to identify research priorities and funding mechanisms and design a peer review system (IOM, 1993).[5] To manage the new breast cancer research program, USAMRMC established a new research area directorate (RAD), now known as the Office of the CDMRP.

---

bill over several years, including $170 million for breast cancer research in FY 1993 (*Congressional Record*, September 16, 1992, p. S13600). The amendment was defeated 62 to 36. The next day, Senator Alphonse D'Amato offered an amendment specifically to transfer $214 million for breast cancer research from DOD to NIH, which was defeated 53-43 (*Congressional Record*, September 17, 1992, p. S13700).

[3]At that time, it was called the U.S. Army Medical Research and Development Command (USAMRDC).

[4]The debate on the amendment, which became Public Law 102-396 on October 6, 1992, is in the *Congressional Record* (September 22, 1992, pp. S14638-S14643). Harkin stated, "Let me make it clear, the Army is not doing this research. The Army is taking this money and they are contracting out to do the research. They can do it with the National Cancer Institute at NIH. They can do it through peer review, and they can have NIH set this up for them" (p. S14640). A member of Harkin's staff told *Nature* magazine that NCI "certainly would provide the most efficient mechanism" for spending the money well (Watson, 1992)

[5]Other accounts of the establishment and early history of CDMRP include Casamayou, 2001:Ch. 6; Stabiner, 1997:Ch. 5; and IOM, 1997:Ch. 4.

At the time, the $210 million constituted a "one-time" appropriation that might or might not be continued in following years (IOM, 1997). The IOM report recommended that at least $151.5 million (72 percent) of the funding should be used for innovative interdisciplinary research projects in the form of new investigator, developmental and exploratory research, and investigator-initiated awards; that up to $27.0 million (13 percent) should be used for training and recruitment fellowships and programs; that up to $21.0 million (10 percent) should be used for infrastructure enhancement, such as banks of tumor samples, tissue, and cell lines and expanded cancer registries; and that $10.5 million (5 percent) should be used for administration (IOM, 1993:Ch. 2).

The report outlined three mechanisms of support for research projects: Individual Investigator Awards (similar to NIH's R01 grants); New Investigator Awards (similar to NIH's R29 FIRST grants); and Innovative Developmental and Exploratory (IDEA) Awards. IDEA Awards were a new mechanism intended to stimulate innovative but high-risk ideas of scientists already in or new to the field of cancer research. These scientists were not required to have the preliminary data that would be required by traditional individual investigator awards. The report recommended that the Army program use a two-tiered review system, in which the first tier would consist of peer review of scientific merit conducted by study sections (i.e., expert panels) and the second tier would consist of an assessment of programmatic relevance by an advisory council of 16 to 18 persons, 3 to 4 of whom would be consumer representatives or representatives of the public interest (IOM, 1993:Ch. 3). The Army adopted the IOM recommendations and engaged the American Institute of Biological Sciences to conduct the peer review process. The 2,668 proposals responding to the Broad Area Announcement issued by USAMRMC in late 1993 were reviewed and scored for scientific merit by 41 peer review panels and were referred to the advisory council recommended by IOM, which was (and still is) called the Integration Panel. The Integration Panel recommended 433 proposals for funding, and the awards were made by the end of September 1994 (Kaiser, 1994).[6]

Evolution of the Program

Few major changes have been made in the structure and administration of the program since the implementation of the FY 1993 appropriation. Consumers were added to the peer review panels in 1995. Additional programs were added, each with its own first tier peer review panels and second tier Integration Panel, following the BCRP model. CDMRP has over time expanded to include seven additional core research programs—neurofibromatosis in FY 1996; prostate cancer and ovarian cancer in FY 1997, biomedical issues directly relevant to military

[6]The review process is described in detail by Schwartz et al., 1995.

health known as the Peer Reviewed Medical Research Program (PRMRP) in FY 1999; and tuberous sclerosis, chronic myelogenous leukemia, and prion disease in FY 2002—each established by Congress at the urging of advocacy groups.[7] Each program has its own peer review panels and Integration Panel composed of scientists, clinicians, health care professionals, and consumer advocates who have extensive knowledge of or experience with the disease in question, or both.

In 1997, IOM was asked to review CDMRP's BCRP. The report of the review noted that, beginning with the FY 1996 program announcements inviting applications, the program underwent a significant shift in program priorities and strategies:

> While formerly oriented toward research on breast cancer prevention, detection, treatment, and quality of life, the mission of the BCRP explicitly shifted towards breast cancer eradication...the mandate to eradicate the disease was to be achieved by emphasis on innovation and new ideas, bringing new investigators into the field, focusing on under-represented areas, and fostering multidisciplinary approaches. (IOM, 1997:55)

The shift in priorities resulted in increased emphasis on IDEA and other award mechanisms for stimulating new ideas and innovative approaches both in basic and translational research. As will be documented below, the emphasis on exploratory research and new investigators has continued up to the present.

Contributions of the Program

IOM's review in 1997 was conducted too early in the program to see research results. The report concluded that USAMRMC had "succeeded in establishing a fair peer review system and a broad-based research portfolio by stimulating scientist from a wide range of disciplines to participate as applicants, reviewers, and advisers" (IOM, 1997:11). It went on to say:

> The [IOM] committee commends the Army for developing such a program under the serious time constraints and fluctuations in funding that have characterized the program to date. Moreover, the program fills a unique niche among public and private funding sources for cancer research. It is not duplicative of other programs and is a promising vehicle for forging new ideas and scientific breakthroughs in the nation's fight against breast cancer.

The 1997 IOM committee identified a number of outstanding program features, including the flexibility of the annual priority setting process; the use of outside peer reviewers to evaluate proposals; the involvement of consumer advocates in the peer review process; and low administrative costs. It called for authorizing the program on a continuing rather than a year-to-year basis; introducing ongoing

---

[7]CDMRP also administered two research programs for one year (FY 1995): osteoporosis and defense women's health.

planning and evaluation; and establishing an outside committee for oversight and program evaluation.

CDMRP had already evaluated the impact of including consumers on peer review panels, finding that technical experts as well as consumers considered consumer involvement to be beneficial (Andejeski et al., 2002a, 2002b). In addition, CDMRP has identified many of the program's contributions in the areas of programmatic innovations, the building of infrastructure, and research advances.

Programmatic Innovations

Innovative program features include the participation of consumer advocates in all aspects of priority setting and peer review; a criteria-based scoring system for reviewing research proposals; and the development of the IDEA Award to foster innovation by supporting higher risk but potentially higher gain research ideas (Young-McCaughan et al., 2002; Rich et al., 1998).

Infrastructure Building

CDMRP has funded the development of shared research resources, such as registries; tissue, tumor, and cultured cell banks; transgenic animals; databases; and research centers and consortia. The cell banks were used in important telomerase studies and in the development of a BRCA1 mutant cell line. The program has also supported the development of new investigators and the involvement of experienced investigators from other fields of research. Through 2002, CDMRP had made more than 1,500 training and recruitment awards, including 35 institutional training grants, 1,156 pre- and postdoctoral fellowships, and 184 career development awards and sabbaticals (CDMRP, 2003:Table II-3).

Research Advances

DOD-funded investigators have made a number of advances. The most notable is probably the identification and understanding of antagonists to the overexpression of the *HER2* gene, which led to the development of Herceptin, a breast cancer therapeutic agent based on an anti-*HER2* antibody (CDMRP, 1999:Section 5). BCRP awarded Dennis Slamon two grants in 1993 totaling $1.7 million to establish a tumor tissue bank and study the biologic effects of *HER2* overexpression and the impact of agonists and antagonists to the *HER2* receptor in human breast tumor normal cell lines.[8] Slamon had begun this work several

---

[8]See abstract of Slamon's proposal at cdmrp.army.mil/scripts/get_item.asp?item=abstract&type=technical&log_no=BC931306 (accessed June 29, 2004) and publications associated with the award at cdmrp.army.mil/scripts/get_item.asp?item=product&type=PUB&log_no=BC931306 (accessed June 29, 2004).

TABLE 1-1 CDMRP Award Results, FY 1993-FY 2003

	BCRP	PCRP	OCRP	NFRP
Publications in Scientific Journals	~6,200	~700	~100	~125
Abstracts/Presentations at Professional Meetings	~4,200	~800	~120	~155
Patents/Licensures (including applications)	~140	~35	~6	6

SOURCE: CDMRP, 2003.

years earlier with funding from the National Cancer Institute and Revlon, but researchers still lacked a regular source of breast tissue from women with breast cancer, women who were high risk (from biopsies), and normal women (from breast reduction surgery) (Stabiner, 1997:410).

Other investigators have studied the function of the hereditary breast cancer gene, BRCAl, and have developed a functional assay for BRCAl that can distinguish between normal and mutant copies of the gene. An early IDEA grant for $148,000 led to the development of FDA-approved devices for conducting ductal lavage, useful in studying cancer of the milk ducts of the breast. The grant recipient, Susan Love, could not obtain funding elsewhere, because she had never done research and her idea was unconventional (Haran, 2001). Prostate Cancer Research Program (PCRP)-funded researchers have discovered three genes implicated in hereditary prostate cancer and another gene that is frequently missing in nonhereditary metastatic prostate cancers, indicating that it might play an important role in suppressing the spread of prostate cancer (CDMRP, 2003:IV-12).

The CDMRP website includes a searchable database of award abstracts and publications associated with them.[9] The number of publications in peer-reviewed journals, abstracts presented at professional meetings, and patents and licenses granted or applied for is in Table 1-1.

Since its inception through FY 2004, CDMRP has managed research programs that have totaled nearly $3 billion in congressional appropriations, and it has awarded a total of 4,910 grants and contracts, with appropriations made for peer reviewed research each year since 1992. Although CDMRP began as an artifact of the budget process in the early 1990s, it has grown to be well respected by the beneficiaries of its programs (advocacy groups and scientists), who view it as efficient, effective, responsive to science, and as a program with relatively low overhead costs (6 percent across core programs).

As new programs were added to CDMRP and the budget escalated—and the call for more earmarked funding grew louder—more organizations began to

[9]See cdmrp.army.mil/scripts/search.asp.

compete for the same pool of funds. However, budgetary constraints have led Congress to question whether funding increases to these programs can continue within the resources available for military spending and whether there might be some way to leverage the investment in these programs through partnerships or collaborations with nonfederal sources.

IMPETUS FOR THIS REPORT

The conference report for DOD's FY 2004 appropriations contained a provision entitled "Cost Sharing for Medical Research Programs," in which it commended DOD "for its management of the peer reviewed medical research and cancer research programs," but noted "with concern the challenge of funding increases to these programs within the resources available for military spending" (U.S. Congress, 2003). The conferees directed "the Assistant Secretary of Defense (Health Affairs), in consultation with the service Surgeons General and the Institute of Medicine, to investigate alternative funding sources, including private sector and non-Federal contributions that can best be used to leverage appropriated funds without biasing the peer review selection process."

In response, the IOM Committee on Alternative Funding Strategies for DOD's Peer Reviewed Biomedical Research Program was established to assess current and alternate funding mechanisms and funding sources, which include private sector and other nonfederal entities, for conducting biomedical research. Specifically, the committee was asked to carry out the following tasks:

1. Advise DOD on how these sources and mechanisms can be leveraged to augment appropriate funds.

2. Identify and advise DOD on new, possible future avenues of funding other than those described in task one.

3. Identify and advise DOD on:
   a. Issues inherent in the federal procurement system that would impact grants and cooperative agreements
   b. Regulations and policies should alternate funding strategies be used.

4. Identify risks and solutions regarding bioethics and peer review bias with respect to alternate funding.

To conduct its assessment in the short period of time allotted, the committee met three times between March and May and convened a two-day workshop April 26-27, 2004, where it heard numerous perspectives on the charge before it. Presenters included stakeholders from voluntary health agencies (VHAs) affiliated with the disease-specific programs of CDMRP, individuals representing public-private partnerships, industrial and other private philanthropic and not-for-profit research sponsors, academic researchers and administrators, and representatives of state-run research programs (see Appendix C for the workshop agenda). In addition, the committee was briefed by CDMRP program managers. Much of the committee's fact-gathering effort was focused on understanding the nature of the CDMRP research programs, which are described below. This understanding provided the backdrop against which any recommendations about alternative or supplemental sources of funding had to be considered.

OVERVIEW OF THE CURRENT CDMRP

CDMRP is a unit of USAMRMC—the medical research, development, logistics, and acquisition arm of the U.S. Army. USAMRMC operates six medical research laboratories and institutes that represent the core science and technology capability of the Command and that serve as centers of excellence in specific areas of biomedical research related to combat medicine.[10] In addition to CDMRP, the Command is organized around four core RADs for infectious diseases, combat casualty care, military operational medicine, and medical chemical and biological defense. There is also a Telemedicine and Advanced Technology Research Center (TATRC).

In addition to the medical research programs planned by the Army, the Command administers programs added to the DOD budget by Congress, called Congressional Special Interest (CSI) programs, not all of which are administered by CDMRP. Some are assigned to the appropriate RAD or to TATRC. Current examples of CSI programs include Military Human Immunodeficiency Virus Research; Surgical Tissue Replacement and Repair; the Neurotoxin Exposure Treatment Program; the Osteoporosis and Bone Health Research Program; Epidermolysis Bullosa Research; and the Center for Innovative Minimally Invasive Therapy.

Partnerships: Consumers, the Scientific Community, and the Military

Most notably, CDMRP has been a pioneer in its work in consumer involvement in scientific priority setting (Rich et al., 1998). The participation of consumer reviewers, who are considered an integral part of the peer review and programmatic processes—and who act as equal partners with scientists—has helped assure that the human dimensions of a disease are incorporated into the scientific and program policy considerations, the investment strategy, and the research focus. Although limited in number, consumer reviewers are full voting members of the peer review panel. DOD works to achieve a broad ethnic and

[10] See mrmc-www.army.mil/.

cultural representation of consumer reviewers by disseminating information to minority consumer groups and by performing formal outreach activities targeted to these groups.

CDMRP makes every attempt to ensure that consumers have an equal voice in all processes, from the initial stakeholders' meeting through programmatic and peer review. Survivors and their family members are well informed and offer a variety of perspectives, with some who focus on basic research, while others demonstrate more knowledge about diagnosis and treatment. Part of the reason that consumer representatives are so well informed is that advocacy groups, such as NBCC, provide training programs to teach consumers about science, as well as lobbying and advocacy.

Scientists and clinicians provide the needed subject matter expertise on peer review panels, and basic scientists and clinicians participate in vision setting and programmatic review, helping CDMRP support innovative, interdisciplinary approaches and collaborations in the scientific community that lead to uncovering the complex causes of disease and translating this knowledge into improvements in disease prevention, patient survival, and quality of life.

Military personnel, civilian, and contractor staff are responsible for executing the congressional directives, working together to implement each program. Several programs have a direct military focus, particularly that of improving the health of the military forces. The military continues to be a central partner in all aspects of CDMRP, through day-to-day coordination and administration, through programs that have a military focus, and through supporting research with the Small Business Innovation Research Program (SBIR).

Representatives of private industry sit on CDMRP Integration Panels, as do members of the public and other funding agencies, such as NCI, the Centers for Disease Control and Prevention (CDC), FDA, and the National Science Foundation, and they participate in discussions regarding effective business processes. In fact, before an Integration Panel is convened, the manager of a particular research program holds a meeting during which the various stakeholders who have an interest in that program can make recommendations. The Ovarian Cancer Research Program meeting, for example, would include representatives of pharmaceutical companies, biotechnology companies, different advocacy groups, NCI, and others who fund ovarian cancer research. These groups also help CDMRP programs establish their initial Integration Panels.

By most accounts, CDMRP has been efficiently managed, scientifically productive, and a valuable component of the nation's health research enterprise, despite initial skepticism about its location in DOD and the participation of consumers in peer review as well as priority-setting processes. Some of the distinctive features of CDMRP are its inclusive program planning and priority-setting process, the rigorous peer review of proposals for scientific merit and program relevance by outside reviewers that includes consumers, the inclusion of VHAs representing patients and survivors in both the priority-setting and peer review processes, the emphasis on exploratory high-risk/high-gain basic, translational, and clinical research projects and research capacity building, and the periodic sharing of results by investigators. Because of the size and focus of the programs, advocacy groups find CDMRP particularly accessible.

At the committee's April workshop, Fran Visco, President of NBCC, said, "It is transparent in large part because it is focused on a particular issue and because of the program structure and the budget limitations. It is functional. It is responsive to real need." Advocates also support the program's strategy of fostering innovation by supporting novel ideas and new investigators. At the time of the establishment of BCRP, the original program, advocates for breast cancer research saw the program as a way to support new ideas about the causes of disease that could be translated into new treatments, instead of supporting research to extend and refine ideas that have been proven, which NIH was already doing with far greater resources (Marshall, 1993). In general, the emphasis on novel ideas and new investigators—whether the research is basic, clinical, or translational—has been adopted by all CDMRP programs.

Funding of CDMRP

In contrast to the individual institutes and centers of NIH, which are legislatively created standing entities that focus consistently on certain key diseases, CDMRP programs depend on yearly congressional appropriations for each program because they are not included in the President's proposed budget for DOD. Congress adds the funds annually to the DOD appropriation to fund new programs or to augment existing DOD or Army programs. Thus, CDMRP originated and operates within an environment that required and fostered the development of novel approaches to its operation as a funding agency.

Planning occurs one year at a time, with no standing peer review panels. This allows CDMRP to create new research opportunities and to focus funding on the most recently recognized research gaps or controversies. The Integration Panel seeks a broad portfolio of grants across all disciplines and often gives preference to those proposals that involve interdisciplinary or collaborative research or that address a program priority, even if this results in funding proposals that may not have received the top score in peer review. Table 1-2 provides a summary of the funding history for each of the existing programs, from 1992 to 2004.[11] Figure 1-1 depicts the planning and funding process of CDMRP.

There are advantages to CDMRP being funded through annual congressional appropriations. Advocates who lobby Congress for funds are invested in the

---

[11]After the report was drafted, Congress passed the FY 2005 appropriations bill for DOD, which continued the core programs at the FY 2004 level except for the Tuberous Sclerosis Complex Research Program ($3.2 million) and the National Prion Research Program ($1.5 million). See thomas.loc.gov/cgi-bin/cpquery/R?cp108:FLD010:@1(hr622).

TABLE 1-2 Funding History of CDMRP Core Programs (in millions of dollars)

Program	FY92	FY93	FY94	FY95	FY96	FY97	FY98	FY99	FY00	FY01	FY02	FY03	FY04
Breast Cancer	25.0	210.0	30.0	150.0	75.0	108.3	135.0	136.8	176.3	177.4	151.5	152.2	150.0
Prostate Cancer						45.0	40.0	50.0	75.0	100.0	85.0	85.0	85.0
Neurofibromatosis					8.0	8.0	9.8	11.5	15.0	17.0	21.0	20.0	20.0
Ovarian Cancer						7.5	10.0	10.0	12.0	12.0	10.2	10.0	10.0
Peer Reviewed Medical Research								19.5	25.0	50.0	50.0	50.0	50.0
Chronic Myelogenous Leukemia											5.0	4.3	4.3
Tuberous Sclerosis Complex											1.0	2.0	3.0
National Prion											42.5	0	0
Total	25.0	210.0	30.0	150.0	83.0	168.8	194.8	227.8	303.3	356.4	366.2	323.5	322.3

SOURCE: Annual reports of CDMRP.

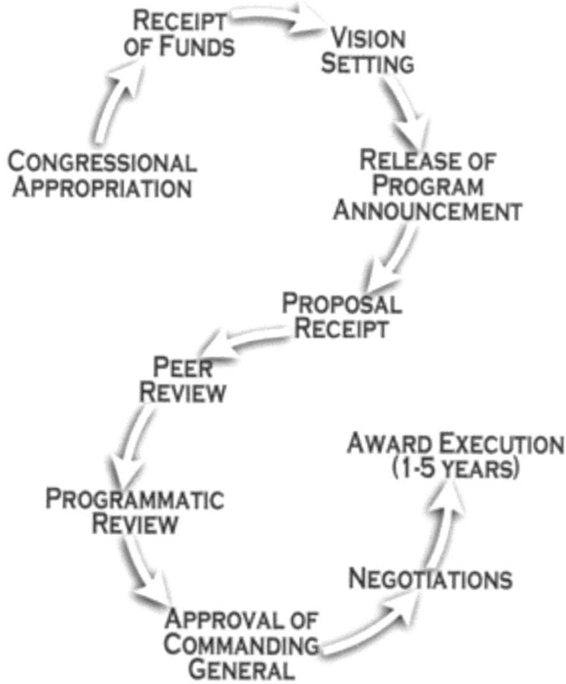
RECEIPT OF FUNDS
VISION SETTING
RELEASE OF PROGRAM ANNOUNCEMENT
PROPOSAL RECEIPT
PEER REVIEW
PROGRAMMATIC REVIEW
APPROVAL OF COMMANDING GENERAL
NEGOTIATIONS
AWARD EXECUTION (1-5 YEARS)
CONGRESSIONAL APPROPRIATION

FIGURE 1-1 CDMRP budget and program planning and execution cycle.
SOURCE: CDMRP, 2003.

program at every level, and the year-to-year funding creates a sense of urgency to fund the best science as quickly as possible. In addition, although there is value in being part of the longer term budget process, the annual appropriations process means that earmarked money is less likely to be involved in a DOD funding rescission. Also, programs can make changes relatively quickly and responsively because they do not have long-term funding commitments. A disadvantage is that it is never known whether a particular program will exist from year to year. CDMRP has two years in which to obligate funds, however, and each award is fully funded up front, which enables the program to support projects of up to five years' duration.

CDMRP Programs

Since its inception, CDMRP has managed 29 separate programs, 8 of which are considered core programs. Core programs have either received or have the potential to receive multiple appropriations and are characterized by standing Integration Panels. The other programs managed by CDMRP have either received a one-time appropriation and/or are institutionally based. Each program emphasizes the specific needs of its research and advocacy communities. The core programs are described in Box 1-1.

BOX 1-1
CDMRP Core Programs

The **Breast Cancer Research Program (BCRP)** is the second largest funder of extramural breast cancer research in the world, having managed approximately $1.52 billion in appropriations from FY 1992 to FY 2003. The awards supported through this program—which attempts to avoid duplicating NIH research funding approaches in this area through a complementary strategy—support innovative ideas, train future generations of scientists and clinicians, provide necessary research resources, bring bench research to the bedside, and emphasize the fostering of research in nontraditional areas for which pilot data may be lacking. Through FY 2002, BCRP has received more than 19,840 proposals and has made 3,671 awards.

The **Chronic Myelogenous Leukemia Research Program (CMLRP)** was established in FY 2002 with a $5 million appropriation for research and was continued in FY 2003 and FY 2004 with congressional appropriations of $4.25 million each year.

The **National Prion Research Program (NPRP)** was established by a one-time congressional appropriation of $42.5 million in FY 2002. The goal of NPRP is to develop a rapid, sensitive, and reproducible test for the detection of prions suitable for use both as an ante-mortem diagnostic test and a screening assay. In support of this goal, additional topics of interest include the prevention, transmission, and pathogenesis of transmissible spongiform encephalopathies as well as a better understanding of chronic wasting disease. A total of 38 awards have been made.

The **Neurofibromatosis Research Program (NFRP)** has managed $110.3 million in congressional appropriations for FY 1996 through FY 2003. In the words of Brenda Duffy, President of Neurofibromatosis, Inc., at the April workshop, "Neurofibromatosis is a very small part of the DOD peer reviewed medical research program. The NF community cannot raise even a fraction of the money that goes to research as a result of the [CDMRP] program." From FY 1996 to FY 2002, NFRP received 299 proposals, leading to 103 awards.

The **Ovarian Cancer Research Program (OCRP)** appropriations for FY 1997 through FY 2003 have totaled $71.7 million. Since the program's inception through

CDMRP Program Planning and Execution

CDMRP has refined over the years a program execution and management strategy that allows it to adapt to the current needs of the research, clinical, and consumer communities. It uses a flexible seven-year execution and management cycle that spans all phases of program execution, from the development of a

September 2003, 575 proposals have been received and 63 awards have been made. Ann Kolker, Ovarian Cancer National Alliance, noted at the April workshop that this federal investment is significant given the scarcity of funds in the private sector, stating that, "given the very, very small amount of privately raised funds available for ovarian cancer research, it is frankly completely unrealistic to expect that charitable foundations and similar organizations could augment in any significant way the investment made by the Federal Government in ovarian cancer research."

The **Peer Reviewed Medical Research Programs (PRMRPs)** supports research on issues with direct relevance to military health. Appropriations for FY 1999 through FY 2002 have totaled $194.5 million. The program has built a research portfolio covering awards that span 32 topic areas relevant to military health. This program uses an advisory panel composed of representatives from the Army, Navy, Air Force, Marines, Department of Veterans Affairs, Office of the Assistant Secretary of Defense (Health Affairs), and U.S. Department of Health and Human Services to develop an investment strategy and conduct programmatic review. In the first four years of the program, 558 proposals have been received and 98 awards have been made.

The **Prostate Cancer Research Program (PCRP)** was established in FY 1997. As a major funder of prostate cancer research, PCRP has been responsible for the management of $480 million in appropriations supporting innovative, multidisciplinary basic and clinical research relevant to prostate cancer. In addition, the program is committed to addressing the significant disparities in the incidence and mortality of prostate cancer that exist among different ethnic groups and has designed award mechanisms to stimulate research in these areas. For the first six years of this program, more than 3,400 proposals have been received, leading to 797 awards.

The **Tuberous Sclerosis Complex Research Program (TSCRP)** was established by a $1 million appropriation in FY 2002 and was continued in FY 2003 and FY 2004 with congressional appropriations of $2 million and $3 million, respectively. TSCRP is supporting innovative research directed toward improving understanding of the role and function of proteins produced by the TSC1 and TSC2 tumor suppressor genes.

vision through the awarding of research grants. Early in each fiscal year, after the congressional appropriation has been signed into law and funds have been received by the USAMRMC, each program's Integration Panel meets to deliberate issues and concerns unique to that program and to establish a vision and investment strategy for the coming year. The investment strategy provides the framework and direction necessary to most effectively obligate each congressional appropriation, while avoiding unnecessary duplication with other funding agencies.

Award Mechanisms

A critical component of the CDMRP investment strategy is the development of specific award mechanisms that capture the current needs of both the research and advocacy communities. Separate announcements outlining the award mechanisms offered for each of the research programs managed by CDMRP are released each fiscal year. CDMRP has employed more than 40 types of award mechanisms, which fall into three categories: research; training and recruitment; and research resources. Awards are made in the form of grants, contracts, or cooperative agreements, with the research executed over one to five years, depending on the type of award mechanism.

Some of the research awards are designed to encourage innovative research by supporting ideas with little or none of the supporting data that the usual investigator-initiated applications must have. These awards have titles such as IDEA, Concept, or Exploratory and are equivalent to such NIH awards as R05 and R21 grants. The proportion of funding going to these awards to test novel ideas is high (more than half [57 percent] in FY 2002), although the percentage varies somewhat from program to program (see Figure 1-2).

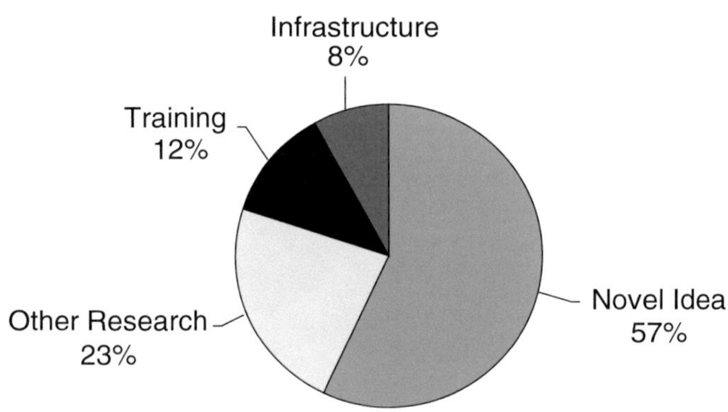

FIGURE 1-2 Distribution of extramural award funding among types of research support, FY 2002.
SOURCE: Calculated from CDMRP, 2003.

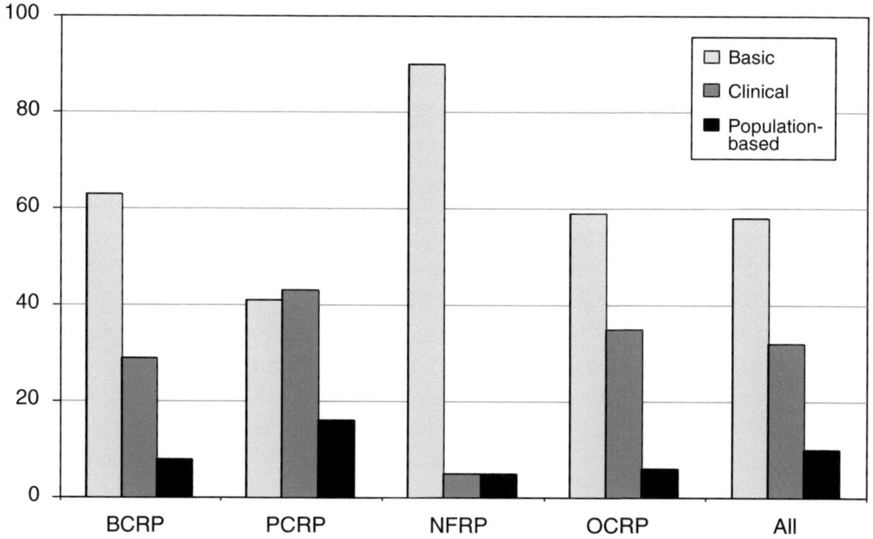

FIGURE 1-3 Distribution of extramural award funding among areas of research, FY 2002 (in percentages).
SOURCE: CDMRP, 2003.

Most of the mechanisms fund either basic or clinical research[12] (e.g., IDEA Awards, New Investigator Awards, and Center Initiation Awards), while other mechanisms support clinical research exclusively (e.g., Clinical Translational Research Awards and Clinical Trial Awards). There also are training mechanisms (Pre- and Postdoctoral Fellowships and Career Development Awards), some of which provide support for investigators at Historically Black Colleges and Universities and Minority Institutions (e.g., Partnership Training Awards). More than half the funding goes to basic research, about a third to clinical research, and a tenth goes to population-based research. Again, the balance varies from program to program (see Figure 1-3). It should be noted that while the percentage of funding going to novel ideas (67 percent) and basic research (68

[12]Basic research is that conducted to increase the base knowledge and understanding of the physical, chemical, and functional mechanisms of life processes and disease. It is fundamental and not directed to solving any particular biomedical problem in humans or animals. This type of research often involves observing, describing, measuring, and conducting experimental manipulation and it provides the basis on which other types of research (applied and clinical) are formed. In contrast, clinical research applies the knowledge gained in basic and applied research to study problems of human disease or dysfunction in a new way. Clinical research generally that takes place in a hospital or clinical setting.

percent) is about the same, they are not congruent. IDEA and similar awards support clinical and translational research as well as basic research.

Each research program has a slightly different group of awards in its portfolio, with the mix depending on how other organizations and agencies are funding research in that area and on the amount of money Congress has appropriated to DOD for research on that disease. Although each award mechanism has different requirements, CDMRP works in all cases to promote innovative research by encouraging investigators to seek out novel, creative ideas, and solutions that will lead to disease-specific research in new directions.

The training and recruitment of new investigators, as well as the building of research resources in the form of centers of excellence, consortia, and imaging equipment, are major investments by CDMRP. For example, training awards are used to train the next generation of cancer investigators, while IDEA Awards, first instituted by BCRP in FY 1996, fund high-risk research projects that have the potential for large breakthroughs. Although IDEA Awards, which have now been adopted by other CDMRP programs, do not generally require the preliminary data that are typically required through other funding mechanisms, but proposals are still expected to be based on sound scientific principles. Thus, IDEA Awards are a critical source of funding for young investigators who lack research data accumulated over a longer career and for investigators who arrive at a novel approach for study.

Nonfederal Cost Sharing

According to CDMRP program announcements that invite applications for research funding, grantee institutions, whether commercial or nonprofit, are expected to "cost share" by providing the equipment needed to support proposed research. In rare cases that are individually negotiated, DOD will pay for 50 percent of the cost of the additional equipment needed to carry out a research project. DOD, however, takes into account the greater need for equipment at Historically Black Colleges and Universities and Minority Institutions.

Examples of Leveraging

There are many examples of CDMRP's work in leveraging resources to facilitate and manage efforts to prevent and cure cancer and other diseases.

Matching Funds and Cost Sharing

In the early years of the prostate cancer program, matching funds were requested from other institutions. Currently, CDMRP has a group of contract specialists and grant managers who serve as technical advisors during award negotiations and work with the institutions to match costs in certain areas. Because matching is not built into program announcements—except in the case of matching funds for equipment—a great deal of this activity takes place in the background. CDMRP also works to implement cost-sharing arrangements. IDEA Awards, for example, provide only $125,000 per year, which is not sufficient for conducting a clinical trial. Cost sharing helps make up the difference and takes place in the form of donations, which can be made for drugs, equipment, and some salaries. Cost sharing also may occur for research-related subject costs, such as blood tests and other components of a clinical trial or human research when these are not budgeted in CDMRP grants.

SBIR Program

CDMRP began participating in the SBIR program under DOD's purview in FY 2000. After programmatic or peer review, if a significant gap remains in submissions or funding is insufficient for the accepted projects, CDMRP will offer an RFP for that area. For example, CDMRP has offered a SBIR RFP for ovarian cancer detection methods and has found this method of leveraging to be worthwhile, as it has recouped about 28 percent of the dollars spent. CDMRP has discussed the use of the SBIR model in some of its programs, particularly in looking at clinical and translation research in clinical trials, with the goal of providing more support in the drug development process, perhaps through Phase I or Phase II.

Examples of Partnerships

A central theme of almost all of the CDMRP award mechanisms is finding and funding the best and most innovative research aimed at eradicating disease. CDMRP programs look for untapped opportunities and underserved areas of research, and in the process they create partnerships and garner public trust. CDMRP investment strategies are re-evaluated annually, with success gauged in part by how many products are brought to the patient. CDMRP's strategy of funding high-risk/high-payoff research means that many ideas do not pan out, but some have, leading quickly to Phase I clinical trials. In some cases, the clinical trials have involved partnerships with other organizations.

- In 2004 CDMRP joined the Gynecological Cancer Foundation Allied Support Group, which includes eight major ovarian cancer funders and 14 advocacy organizations. CDMRP works to facilitate synergy among these organizations, which share the CDMRP goals of prevention, detection, and education among patients, laypersons, and physicians, particularly primary care physicians.
- In an effort sponsored by BCRP, CDMRP is collaborating with the National Society of Nursing Oncologists to increase consumer participation in clinical trials, particularly those for gynecological diseases. The Era of Hope meeting

includes representatives from industry, public funding agencies, private funding agencies, and Historically Black Colleges and Universities and Minority Institutions, as well as survivors, scientists, clinicians, lawyers, and ethicists, to discuss not only DOD research findings, but also the use of innovation, invention, creativity, and collaboration to move findings from the bench to the bedside quickly.

- CDMRP has co-funded grants with the National Cancer Institute, Office of the NIH Director, Department of Health and Human Services Office on Women's Health, and California Breast Cancer Research Program.
- PRMRP currently is holding a health research forum where program investigators and others instrumental in DOD-related research can discuss collaborations and strategies for progress.
- NPRP has collaborated with numerous agencies throughout the country and will continue to hold meetings and form partnerships with others.

Communication with Other Funding Agencies and the Public

CDMRP's use of the Common Scientific Outline (CSO) reflects its support for improved communication among funding agencies in the United States and abroad. This outline was initiated by NCI to categorize its funded research projects in a scientific and disease-related manner with the goal of reducing duplication and facilitating complementary research. CDMRP was invited to participate in this effort in 1997 and worked with NCI to develop a working model of the CSO. In subsequent years, additional cancer-funding organizations were asked to join the efforts of NCI and CDMRP in evaluating the utility of the CSO as a tool to facilitate the description of their respective portfolios and communication among funders. The CSO now includes 9 major cancer funders from the United States and 15 from the United Kingdom. In addition, CDMRP recently increased its effort to increase public awareness of its programs through advertising specific award mechanisms in national newspapers, distributing award information to consumer advocacy groups, and sponsoring funded investigators to attend scientific meetings.

More than 4,500 publications have resulted from CDMRP awards through FY 2001 and CDMRP staff has published articles and presented information at national scientific meetings. In addition, the CDMRP website disseminates up-to-date program information to the public and research community, and programs prepare and issue program announcements that provide details on individual award mechanisms, the application process, and requirements for submitting proposals.

THE COMMITTEE'S APPROACH TO ITS TASK

Over the course of its deliberations, the committee did not systematically evaluate CDMRP and its outcomes or compare its programs directly with those of NIH or any other federal funding agency. Not only was such an evaluation outside its charge, but it also would have required far more time than was permitted. In general, the committee, based on testimony provided by advocacy groups and members of the scientific community at the April workshop, and committee members' own knowledge of the program, supported the view that the CDRMP programs are of high quality and should be maintained. Rather than question those assumptions, it responded to its charge to identify potential sources of nonfederal funding, identify the range of mechanisms that could be used to leverage that nonfederal funding, and evaluate the impacts that the various potential mechanisms might have on the current program.

An important task of the committee was to define "leveraging." In the federal grants world, the concept of leveraging retains the general idea that more is gained than invested (Feller, 1997:32-33). In one common type of leveraging, the agency is attempting to extend program funding to be able to make more research awards. This is typically achieved by imposing cost sharing or matching requirements on awardees. Another type of leveraging involves using federal awards to encourage other funders to collaborate in ways that achieve greater or faster results for society, for example, through the creation of synergies, critical mass, economies of scale or scope, or assembly of interdependent inputs (e.g., expertise, databases, research tools) required to tackle a problem. These benefits are the fundamental basis for research partnerships, alliances, and cooperative R&D ventures (Austin, 2000:8-10). The parties willingly collaborate to produce results that could not be reached if each acted alone—or at least not reached as quickly or easily. Companies, for example, might agree to jointly fund research that no one of them could afford to do alone and from which all could benefit.

The committee discussed another aspect of leveraging—that is, whether the nonfederal resources that are leveraged are new. New resources are those that otherwise would have been allocated to another purpose than research. Leveraging new resources increases the size of the funding pie, while leveraging funds that would have been spent on related research simply reallocates the resources included in the existing pie. Although a funding agency may claim it has increased funding for its research program, it may in fact have merely shifted funding from equivalent uses. Shifting funds in this way results in little or no net benefit, unless of course the recombined resources permit the attainment of an important result that could not otherwise be achieved.

The committee views leveraging that is intended to increase research results as preferable to leveraging that is intended simply to extend program funding, because the latter tends to shift funding without increasing social benefit. This position is consistent with recent federal policy changes regarding cost sharing, which will be discussed in Chapter 4. On the other hand, using CDMRP funds to induce collaborations that result in the whole becoming greater than the sum of the parts would clearly be beneficial and should be encouraged.

Although the committee was cognizant of the political pressures exerted on Congress to expand what is believed to be a successful program, it recognized that funding decisions are congressional responsibilities and that citizens have the right to petition their government for federal support of such programs. The committee was not asked to comment on this dynamic, which was central to the creation and expansion of CDMRP. Although there is widespread support of CDMRP from advocacy groups and much of the scientific community, committee members are aware that some of their colleagues in the policy and scientific communities view the program with some degree of skepticism because of its location in the federal government outside NIH and the circumstances by which it was created.

During its deliberations the committee was cognizant of the changing funding environment for biomedical research. Since the creation of CDMRP, the NIH budget has doubled over a five-year period, and increasing demands have been placed on the overall DOD budget. Although these events were not central to its analysis, the committee considered them to be important trends when viewing CDMRP in a larger context.

In addition, the committee noted the importance of viewing the federal biomedical research investment in its entirety when making funding decisions, which means considering the breadth and depth of programs supported by other federal agencies, such as the Department of Veterans Affairs, NIH, and CDC. However, the committee was asked to focus more specifically on nonfederal sources of funding to augment CDMRP, rather than on similar federally funded programs where collaboration and leveraging also might be achieved.

One of the main tasks that faced the committee involved assessing whether and how changes made to bring private or nonfederal funds into the program would affect the positive contributions the program is currently making, a view that could be characterized as "first, do no harm." This approach could also be characterized as an analysis of the tradeoffs between bringing more money into the program to fund a greater amount of research versus the cost of the changes that would be needed in order to gain those financial resources. Each potential source of alternative funding was assessed with these concerns in mind. The committee considered whether federal rules and regulations would have to be revised to address bioethical concerns or peer review biases that might result from collaborative funding mechanisms or from the infusion of nonfederal funds into the DOD programs.

Chapter 2 of this report focuses on sources of nonfederal funding, summarizing the statistics on funding of biomedical research by sector (industry, academia, other nonprofits, venture capital, and state government) and describing their different but complementary goals. This chapter reflects the factual basis for the committee's findings and recommendations concerning *sources* of nonfederal funding.

Chapter 3 identifies and analyzes potential mechanisms for fund raising, based on a typology developed by the committee—that is, through partnerships, cost sharing or matching provisions, challenge grants, piggybacking arrangements, jointly funded research subsidiaries, recoupment or return on investment provisions, or supplemental funding. This chapter describes the factual basis for the committee's findings and recommendations concerning *mechanisms* of non-federal funding.

Chapter 4 provides the committee's analysis of the pros and cons of alternative mechanisms in terms of a common set of criteria or questions, including the three issues mentioned in the charge (federal rules and regulations that might have to be revised, bioethical concerns, and peer review bias) and additional criteria, such as impacts on the distinctive features of the program (consumer participation in priority setting and peer review, annual priority setting, program balance, and low overhead), and the added costs of fundraising.

Finally, Chapter 5 provides the committee's conclusions and recommendations.

REFERENCES

Andejeski Y, Breslau ES, Hart E, Lythcott N, Alexander L, Rich I, Bisceglio I, Smith HS, Visco FM, and the US Army Medical Research and Materiel Command Fiscal Year 1995 Breast Cancer Research Program Integration Panel. 2002a. "Benefits and Drawbacks of Including Consumer Reviewers in the Scientific Merit Review of Breast Cancer Research." *Journal of Women's Health & Gender-Based Medicine*, 11(2):119-136.

Andejeski Y, Bisceglio IT, Dickerson K, Johnson JE, Robinson SI, Smith HS, Visco FM, Rich IM. 2002b. "Quantitative Impact of Including Consumers in the Scientific Review of Breast Cancer Research Proposals." *Journal of Women's Health & Gender-Based Medicine*, 11(4):379-388.

Austin JE. 2000. *The Collaboration Challenge, How Nonprofits and Businesses Succeed through Strategic Alliances*. San Francisco, CA: Jossey-Bass Publishers.

Casamayou MH. 2001. *The Politics of Breast Cancer*. Washington, DC: Georgetown University Press.

CDMRP (Congressionally Directed Medical Research Programs). 1999. *FY99 CDMRP Annual Report*. Fort Detrick, MD: CDMRP. [On-line.] Available: cdmrp.army.mil/annreports/1999annrep/ [accessed May 24, 2004].

CDMRP. 2003. *Department of Defense Congressionally Directed Medical Research Programs: Annual Report*, September 30, 2003. Fort Detrick, MD: Congressionally Directed Medical Research Programs. [On-line.] Available: cdmrp.army.mil/annreports/2003annrep/ [accessed May 24, 2004].

Feller I. 1997. *Matching Fund and Cost-Sharing Experiences of U.S. Research Universities: Final Report to the National Science Foundation*. Bethesda, MD: COSMOS Corporation.

Haran C. 2001. "Three's Company: The Army, Women with Cancer and the Medical Community Have Joined Forces." *MAMM*, 3:38-43,57. [On-line.] Available: cdmrp.army.mil/pubs/articles/threescompany.htm

IOM (Institute of Medicine). 1993. *Strategies for Managing the Breast Cancer Research Program: A Report to the U.S. Medical Research and Development Command*. Washington, DC: National Academy Press.

IOM. 1997. *A Review of the Department of Defense's Program for Breast Cancer Research*. Washington, DC: National Academy Press.

Kaiser J. 1994. "Army Doles Out Its First $210 Million." *Science*, 266(October 14):212.

Marshall E. 1993. "The Politics of Breast Cancer." *Science*, 259(January 29):616-617.

Mervis J. 1993. "U.S. Army to Use Peer Review in Breast Cancer Programme." *Nature*, 363(May 20):195.

Rich IM, Andejeski Y, Alciati MH, Bisceglio IC, Breslau ES, McCall L, Valadez A. 1998. "Perspective from the Department of Defense Breast Cancer Research Program." *Breast Disease*, 10(5,6):33-45.

Schwartz SM, Slater DW, Heydrick FP, Woollett GR. 1995. "A Report of the AIBS Peer-review process for the U.S. Army's 1994 Breast Cancer Initiative." *BioScience*, 45(September):558-563.

Science. 1992. "Army Cancer Chief Gives NIH a Cold Shoulder." *Science*, 258(December 4):1567.

Stabiner K. 1997. *To Dance with the Devil: The New War on Breast Cancer: Politics, Power, and People*. New York, NY: Delacorte Press.

U.S. Congress, House of Representatives, Committee on Appropriations. 2003. H. Rpt. 108-283 (September 24):336-337.

Visco F. 2004. Interview with Fran Visco by Michael McGeary and Rick Erdtmann, at the Institute of Medicine, Washington, DC, February 17.

Washington Fax. 1992. "Extramural Community Will Have the Opportunity to Participate in DOD $210 million Breast Cancer Research Program." Washington DC, December 18. [On-line.] Available: www.washingtonfax.com/p1/1992/19921218.html.

Watson T. 1992. "Congress Supports Breast Cancer Research by Taking $210 Million from Military." *Nature*, 359(October 8):471.

Young-McCaughan S, Rich IM, Lindsay GC, and Bertram KA 2002. "The Department of Defense Congressionally Directed Medical Research Program: Innovations in the Federal Funding of Biomedical Research." *Clinical Cancer Research*, 8(4):957-962.

2

Sources of Funding for Biomedical Research

Biomedical research and development (R&D) is a large enterprise in the United States. In fiscal year (FY) 1999, the last year for which comprehensive survey data are available, federal spending on health R&D was $15.7 billion—21 percent of all federal expenditures on R&D that year (NIH, 2004a). Those figures are much larger in 2004, if only because the budget of the National Institutes of Health (NIH)—which supports roughly 83 percent of federally funded biomedical research—doubled between FY 1998 and FY 2003 and currently stands at more than $28.0 billion. The other major funders of biomedical research are the for-profit pharmaceutical, biotechnology, and medical equipment industries, which have outspent NIH in recent years. The Pharmaceutical Research and Manufacturers of America (PhRMA) reported that in 2003 its member companies (which include most of the large biotechnology companies as well as all the major pharmaceutical companies) spent $27.4 billion on R&D performed in the United States and another $5.8 billion on R&D performed abroad (PhRMA, 2004).

Other funders include venture capital funds; colleges and universities; non-profit research institutions, foundations and other philanthropic and charitable organizations; and state governments. These sources of support are much smaller than the federal government and industry, and because of their small size, they often pursue a strategy of leveraging other resources to achieve their mission.

This chapter reviews the sources of funding that could potentially augment appropriated funds for the Congressionally Directed Medical Research Programs (CDMRP) of the Department of Defense (DOD) and briefly describes the types of R&D activities supported by these sources. Chapter 3 reviews examples of collaborations between the federal and nonfederal funders of research described in this chapter.

THE FEDERAL GOVERNMENT

NIH last conducted a survey of federal support for health R&D in 1999 (NIH, 2004a).[1] In that year, total federal spending on health R&D was approximately $15.7 billion, with NIH the top funder at $13.0 billion (83 percent). Other agencies in the Department of Health and Human Services (DHHS), including the Centers for Disease Control and Prevention (CDC) and the Food and Drug Administration, spent another $758.0 million. Non-DHHS federal agencies—primarily DOD, the Department of Veterans Affairs, and the Department of Energy—spent an additional $1.8 billion. Table 2-1 lists the agencies and their R&D budget obligations for FY 1997 through FY 1999.

Most of the federal funding of health R&D in 1999 was performed by nonfederal research institutions through extramural grants, cooperative agreements, and contracts, with extramural performers accounting for 76 percent of federal expenditures on health R&D. Of the total $11.9 billion spent on extramural health R&D in 1999, institutions of higher education received $8.3 billion, other nonprofits $2.3 billion, industry $0.9 billion, and state and local governments $141.0 million (NIH, 2004b). The NIH survey does not break out the amounts of these funds that go to basic versus applied research.

In 1999, 61 percent of federal expenditures in these fields were classified as basic research and 39 percent as applied research (the National Science Foundation [NSF] survey does not break out development expenditures by field). The emphasis on basic research was primarily due to NIH, which accounted for nearly 90 percent of all basic research funding in the three fields. NIH is the single largest funder of biomedical and behavioral research, with nearly two-thirds of its funding of research projects and centers supporting basic research. Most of the other agencies are mission oriented and place a greater emphasis on applied research and development. As a group, they spent 37 percent of their funding in these fields on basic research. DOD spends nearly three-quarters of its funding of biomedical and behavioral research on applied projects; basic research accounts for 26 percent.

The picture has no doubt changed since 1999, the first year of the five-year doubling of the NIH budget. For FY 2004, the NIH budget is $28.0 billion,[2] and if the other agencies increased funding for health R&D by just 10 percent overall

---

[1]A survey of federal agency funding of health R&D for the years FY 2000 through FY 2002 (actual) and FY 2003 through FY 2004 (estimated) was in the field while this report was being written. The QRC Division of Macro International Inc., is conducting the survey for NIH.

[2]See www4.od.nih.gov/officeofbudget/FY05pubs/MechanismTotal.pdf.

TABLE 2-1 Federal Obligations for Health R&D by Source, FY 1997-FY 1999 (in millions of dollars)

	1997	1998	1999
Department of Health and Human Services	12,676.0	13,575.8	13,812.9
National Institutes of Health	11,993.0	12,880.2	13,005.7
Centers for Disease Control and Prevention	323.0	344.0	433.3
Food and Drug Administration	158.6	142.9	130.3
Health Resources and Services Administration	13.1	11.0	11.6
Office of the Assistant Secretary for Health/ Agency for Healthcare Research and Quality	144.0	146.5	182.3
Other Health and Human Services Agencies	44.3	51.2	49.7
Other Departments and Agencies	2,404.8	2,712.6	1,845.7
Department of Agriculture	127.2	140.1	148.7
Department of Defense*	1,094.2	1,251.7	387.4
Department of Education	24.1	29.1	0
Department of Energy	318.8	367.6	372.2
Environmental Protection Agency	123.5	155.5	141.6
Agency for International Development	32.1	72.3	70.9
National Aeronautics and Space Administration	179.4	174.9	186.4
National Science Foundation	81.1	76.0	81.1
Department of Veterans Affairs	259.9	294.4	294.4
All other departments and agencies	164.6	151.0	162.9
Total	15,080.8	16,288.4	15,658.6

*In FY 1999 DOD funds decreased substantially from estimated amounts because of reallocations.
SOURCE: grants.nih.gov/grants/award/research/sourfund.htm.

since 1999, the total federal investment in health R&D would be nearly $31.0 billion. As already noted, most of this supports extramural awards to institutions of higher education. A small portion is spent in federal, industrial, and state laboratories.

Funding Through Foundations Established for Federal Agencies

One mechanism for expanding the federal government's capacity to fund research is through the creation of foundations, such as the Foundation for the National Institutes of Health (FNIH) or the CDC Foundation (Box 2-1). These independent nonprofit enterprises were created to secure private funding for their agency's activities and facilitate programmatic partnerships between their agency and other organizations—corporations, foundations, other nonprofits, and other government agencies—in efforts to improve public health and safety. They have supported initiatives such as fellowship programs, training, infrastructure, and basic and applied research.

BOX 2-1
The CDC Foundation

The CDC Foundation was established in 1992 by Congress to forge partnerships with CDC to boost the agency's programs. As an independent nonprofit organization, the foundation can accept funding and create programs that help donors and CDC scientists achieve common goals. It can find funding partners, negotiate deals, hire people, manage program budgets, identify experts, and report to donors.

In 2002-2003 the foundation had revenues of $17.1 million and expenses of $10.2 million, of which $8.1 million were expended through cost-reimbursement agreements for programs.

On its website, the foundation currently lists 37 corporations and 23 foundations that were supporting programs initiated as of July 2000 or that are currently active. Listed are 22 Global Health Programs, including:

Asian Rotavirus Surveillance Program – Phase II. Partners: GlaxoSmithKline, PATH (Program for Appropriate Technology in Health)
Development of Rapid Assessment Methods and Tools for Displaced Persons. Partner: Andrew W. Mellon Foundation.
Joint Global Field Epidemiology and Laboratory Training Program–Kenya. Partner: Ellison Medical Foundation.
Lilly International Laboratory Fellowships. Partner: Eli Lilly and Company.
Violent Injury Surveillance and Prevention Program. Partners: John D. and Catherine T. MacArthur Foundation, World Health Organization.

Also listed were eight Promoting Healthy Lifestyles programs, such as:

Avon-CDC Foundation Mobile Access Program. Partner: Avon Foundation
Price Fellowships for HIV Prevention Leadership. Partner: Price Foundation.
Promoting Better Health for Young People Through Physical Activity and Sports. Partner: MetLife Foundation.

The 22 Research and Education Programs included:

Antimicrobial Resistant Bacteria Educational Program. Partners: AB Biodisk; Abbott Laboratories; Becton Dickinson and Company; bioMérieux, Inc.; Dade Microscan, Inc.; Merck & Co., Inc.; Ortho-McNeil Pharmaceutical, Inc.; Roche; GlaxoSmithKline.
Applied Epidemiology Training Program for Medical Students. Partner: Pfizer Inc.
Estimation of Prevalence of Erectile Dysfunction in the U.S. Partners: National Foundation for Sexual Health Medicine, Inc.; Pfizer Inc.

PRIVATE INDUSTRY

Several sources of information are available on industry investment in health and medical research. PhRMA, which includes most of the large biotechnology companies as well as all of the major pharmaceutical companies, annually surveys its member companies on this topic. In 2003, member companies reported that they spent $27.4 billion on R&D performed in the United States and another $5.8 billion on R&D performed abroad (PhRMA, 2004). The total investment of $33.2 billion equaled 17.7 percent of the industry's domestic sales on R&D—a higher percentage than was reported for any other U.S. industry.[3] Like the pharmaceutical industry, the U.S. biotechnology industry is very research-intensive, spending $15.7 billion on research and development in 2001.[4]

The medical equipment and supplies industry and the health care services industry also invest their own funds in R&D ($3.7 billion and $0.5 billion, respectively, in 2000) (NSF, 2003a:Table A-8). Some of this is no doubt spent in areas of CDMRP programs, especially in cancer. In 2003, for example, 181 biotechnology and pharmaceutical companies had nearly 400 medicines for cancer in clinical trials, including 47 for breast cancer, 27 for ovarian cancer, 38 for leukemia, and 44 for prostate cancer (PhRMA, 2003). The only figure for spending by PhRMA members on cancer research is for 1997, when companies reported spending $1.4 billion on cancer R&D, approximately 7.4 percent of total pharmaceutical R&D (PhRMA, 1997). If cancer research continued to constitute 7.4 percent of pharmaceutical R&D (and it was probably more), it would have totaled nearly $2.5 billion in 2003.

The bulk of industrial R&D is conducted in-house on product development. In 2000, for example, the pharmaceuticals and medicines industry and medical equipment and supplies industry spent 84 percent of their R&D budgets in their own laboratories (NSF, 2003a:Table A-10), and most of the rest was contracted to other commercial firms. However, industry also lets contracts and awards grants for R&D at universities. Universities reported receiving $2.2 billion from all industry sectors in 2002 (it is not possible to break out specific industries, such as pharmaceuticals), which together constituted 6 percent of university expenditures on R&D (NSF, 2004b:Table 1).

The advocacy organization Research!America (R!A) generates an estimate of industry funding of health research based on data from PhRMA and the Biotechnology Industry Organization (BIO), adjusted to eliminate the overlap between the organizations' memberships. R!A estimates that pharmaceutical and

---

[3]See www.phrma.org/issues/researchdev/.

[4]See www.bio.org/speeches/pubs/er/statistics.asp. This total overlaps with the total reported by PhRMA, because of double counting of larger biotechnology companies in the two categories of biotechnology and pharmaceutical companies.

biotechnology industries' investments in R&D totaled $45.9 billion in 2001 and $49.9 billion in 2002 (R!A, 2003, 2004).

NSF conducts an annual survey of industrial R&D that reports data by type of industry. In 2000, the pharmaceuticals and medicines industry reported company-funded R&D expenditures of $12.9 billion, the medical equipment and supplies industry $3.8 billion, and health care services $0.6 billion, for a total of $17.2 billion (NSF, 2003a). Of this, approximately $2.7 billion was contracted to outside organizations, including universities. These numbers changed rather dramatically in 2001, when company-funded R&D expenditures totaled $10.1 billion for the pharmaceuticals and medicines industry (a drop of 21 percent), $5.9 billion for the medical equipment and supplies industry (up 57 percent), and $1.1 billion for the health care services industry (up 96 percent) (NSF, 2004a).

As would be expected, industry provides little funding directly to the federal government—approximately $16.1 million through FNIH and additional funding through the CDC Foundation.[5] Industry also provides funding as cost sharing on grants and contracts to universities (the latter amount is unknown, although NSF reported making awards that included cost sharing totaling $534.0 million in FY 2001 (NSF, 2002). Industry collaboration with government is far more likely to occur when a company sees an opportunity to leverage the federal investment in long-term basic research by completing the applied work and development activities necessary to take a product to market.

Although industry invests heavily in biomedical research, it focuses mostly on short-term research and development projects with commercial promise, such as drug development and the creation of research tools and databases that can be used in applied research and development. Industry does, however, invest in some basic research. Most observers estimate that approximately 10 percent of biopharmaceutical industry investment is in basic research, which would amount to from $3 billion to $4 billion per year. If industry R&D investment in cancer research is $2.5 billion annually, 10 percent would amount to $250 million. However, hard, documented figures are not available.

VENTURE CAPITAL

Most venture capital is invested in start-up companies that have the potential to become economically successful—that is, companies that represent an opportunity for a high rate of return within five to seven years. It is an important source of equity for new, fast-growing companies (NVCA, 2004a). According to the MoneyTree survey for the first quarter of 2004, the life sciences sector—which includes companies in biotechnology and medical devices—continued to domi-

[5]In FY 2003, the CDC Foundation expended $8.1 million on programs and projects. The funds were provided by more than 30 companies and 20 foundations.

TABLE 2-2 Expenditures for Biomedical and Behavioral R&D at Universities and Colleges, FY 2001 (dollars in thousands)

Field	Nonfederal	Federal	Total
Biological Sciences	2,071,446	3,872,150	5,943,596
Medical Sciences	3,928,069	6,248,659	10,176,728
Psychology	183,762	398,103	581,865
Total	6,183,277	10,518,912	16,702,189

SOURCE: NSF, 2003b.

nate other industries in winning venture capital (NVCA, 2004b). During the quarter, 27 percent (or $1.3 billion) of total venture capital was invested in 71 biotechnology companies and 51 medical device companies. Proportionately, biotechnology and medical devices accounted for 20 percent and 7 percent, respectively, of all venture capital investments. In general, the goal of venture capital firms is to assist companies in the development of new products or services, not to invest in basic research.

ACADEMIA

NSF also conducts an annual survey of R&D expenditures by colleges and universities that includes data on the source of R&D funds in aggregate, not by field. In FY 2001, the most recent year for which data are available, colleges and universities spent $32.7 billion on R&D, about half of which ($16.7 billion) was spent on the biologic and medical sciences and psychology (NSF, 2003b). Table 2-2 separates these figures by field and by whether the funding was provided by federal or nonfederal sources. Overall, the federal government provided 59 percent ($19.2 billion) of R&D funding, and industry provided 7 percent ($2.2 billion). Colleges and universities reported funding 20 percent ($6.6 billion) from institutional funds. Institutional funds are:

> funds, including related indirect costs, that an institution spends for R&D activities from the following unrestricted sources: general-purpose state or local government appropriations; general-purpose awards from industry, foundations, or other outside sources; tuition and fees; endowment income; gifts; and other institutional funds. (NSF, 2003b:266)

The rest came from state and local governments (7 percent) and other sources (7 percent).

A preliminary NSF report relying on FY 2002 data does not detail expenditures by field, but shows that the distribution of funding sources was about the same as in previous years, including 20 percent ($7.1 billion) from institutional sources (NSF, 2004b). Other data sources report that the federal government accounted for 62 percent of the support awarded to U.S. universities, hospitals, and research institutes between 1991 and 2002 (AUTM, 2002). It is not known, however, how much of this funding was already cost shared or how much more might have been expended from an institution's own funds—such as tuition and fees or endowment income—if required to increase cost sharing.

PHILANTHROPIC ORGANIZATIONS

It is estimated that philanthropic giving totaled about $240 billion in 2003, an increase over 2002 of 0.5 percent after inflation. Individuals by far contributed the largest portion of charitable dollars ($179 billion), most of which went to religious institutions. Corporations donated $13 billion to charity, foundations donated $26 billion, and charitable bequests totaled $22 billion (AAFRC, 2004).

Charitable giving from individuals, companies, foundations, and bequests has increased substantially (94.1 percent) since 1995, but most of this increase occurred before 2000. The compound rate of growth from 1995 to 2000 was 13.0 percent per year; from 2000 to 2003 it was 1.8 percent. Corporate giving has grown at a slower rate than the overall average. Among foundations, large independent (versus corporate, operating, and community) foundations do most of the giving, in 2001 contributing about $23.7 billion, or about 80 percent, of total foundation dollars.

Foundations and public charities such as the American Cancer Society have limited resources compared with the federal government—with foundations contributing $1 billion to $2 billion per year to health research—and most focus on funding activities that are not well supported by the federal government, such as public health, or activities that leverage federal funding, such as grants for exploratory research and new investigators. A few foundations, such as the Juvenile Diabetes Research Foundation International (JDRF), collaborate with federal agencies on projects of mutual interest, but the amounts of money they provide are modest relative to federal funding.

The amount of money provided by private foundations for national health research and development remained fairly constant from 1987 to 1996, but represented a small portion of overall funding. Foundations, voluntary agencies, and the Howard Hughes Medical Institute (HHMI) provided only about 9 percent of the total funding for academic health centers in 1997.

Although many boards of such private organizations will not donate money to a government agency for medical research, they will act as a partner in such efforts. The Burroughs Wellcome Fund, for example, partnered with DOD, the National Institute of Allergy and Infectious Diseases, and the Wellcome Trust on the malaria genome sequencing project. In this case, in addition to providing the dollars to sequence the genome, Burroughs Wellcome provided the top-down steering to bring the research community together on a recurring basis, which helped to provide the community with the tools it needed to accomplish the effort. To be successful in this kind of endeavor—which leverages not only dollars but also expertise and organizational focus—at least one organization has to be the engine that moves the effort forward.

Health foundations that have been created from the proceeds of the sale of nonprofits that are going for-profit are a relatively new source of potential funding, with assets of about $8.0 billion and making grants totaling about $340.0 annually, generally in support of underserved populations. Although their grant making for the most part has not included medical research, these groups potentially could allocate a significant portion of their dollars to such efforts, particularly as related to underserved populations.

HHMI, with assets of close to $11.3 billion in 2003, is not classified as a foundation (it is a medical research organization), but it has a large cadre of elite investigators (who are employees not grantees of the institute), as well as a new research facility, and it provides grants to support life sciences education and research opportunities for K-12 and undergraduate students.

The Foundation Center collects data on patterns of giving by these organizations, with the latest figures included in the 2004 edition of its annual report, *Foundation Giving Trends* (Foundation Center, 2004). In 2002, total grant commitments by participating foundations were $15.9 billion. The largest number of grants and grant dollars were in education and health (Figure 2-1), with "health" defined in the report as including grants to hospitals for medical care.

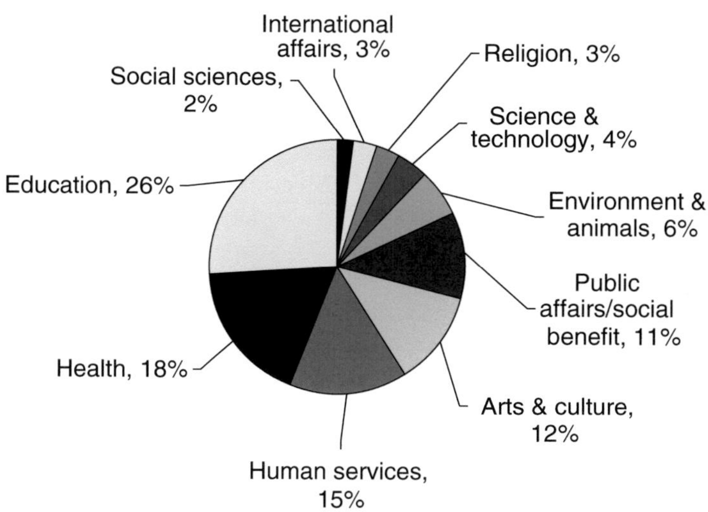

FIGURE 2-1 Foundation grant dollars by purpose, 2002.
SOURCE: Foundation Center, 2004. Based on a sample of 1,005 larger foundations.

TABLE 2.3 The 12 Largest VHAs in Research Grant Expenditures, FY 2002

Association	Grant expenditures (million $)	Percentage of agency budget
American Heart Association	126.2	24
Juvenile Diabetes Research Foundation	107.9	64
American Cancer Society	95.7	11
Cystic Fibrosis Foundation	51.6	36
The Leukemia & Lymphoma Society	37.6	24
Multiple Sclerosis Foundation	32.1	18
American Diabetes Association	31.5	17
March of Dimes	27.7	13
Muscular Dystrophy Association	26.4	17
Arthritis Foundation	25.7	20
Alzheimer's Association	17.5	—
American Lung Association	11.6	7
Total	591.5	—

SOURCE: Lichtman et al., 2004, Table 1.

Most public charities that support medical research are voluntary health agencies (VHAs), which raise a substantial portion of dollars from the public, but may also seek foundation support. VHAs allocate substantial dollars for research; for example, the 12 largest health VHAs spent nearly $600.0 million on research in FY 2002 (Table 2-3). Overall, more than $500 million per year is contributed by some of the larger voluntary organizations to the medical research arena. Many of these VHAs focus their research efforts on a specific disease.

The National Health Council, a nonprofit whose mission is to advance the voluntary health movement and promote the importance of medical research, has more than 45 volunteer agencies as members,[6] and in FY 2000 spent $506.9 million on research, ranging from $4,000 (Myositis Association of America) to $133,562,000 (American Heart Association) annually.

The amount of individual giving going to support medical research is not known, although press releases announcing some large awards and medical school annual reports indicate that a number of gifts are directed annually toward the support of health research—and the amount could be substantial (Bond et al., 1999).[7] It must be remembered, though, that many of these are one-time gifts rather than continuing sources of collaboration and support.

There is no way to know how much collaboration exists between foundations and public charities and federal programs that fund biomedical research. How-

[6]See www.nationalhealthcouncil.org.

[7]See www.aaas.org/spp/cstc/pne/pubs/fundscience/abstracts.htm#bond.

ever, such collaborations do occur, some of which are described in Chapters 3 and 4 and in Appendix A. (Box 2-2 illustrates an example of a foundation that regularly co-funds or coordinates funding of research projects research with NIH.)

Testimony at the committee's April 2004 workshop indicated that philanthropic organizations are changing the focus of their research investment from basic research to clinical, translational, and behavioral research. Although the contribution of such organizations is small compared to federal and industry support, these organizations are always looking for opportunities to leverage their modest dollars, and these dollars are important because they can provide critical "venture capital."[8] Many efforts focus on exploratory research and new investigators, enabling these groups to gather the data needed to support an application for an R01 or similar grant from NIH. Philanthropic organizations often can move quickly to fill a gap, but sometimes they are limited in their ability to provide sustained research support. In addition, they must ensure that research investments are consistent with the charter or mandate of the organization, which might restrict funds geographically or institutionally (Bond et al., 1999).

STATE GOVERNMENTS

State funding for biomedical research has been on the rise since the late 1970s, although most states have had to dramatically cut budgets in recent years as fiscal constraints have worsened (McNichol and Harris, 2004). The National Conference of State Legislatures estimates that since FY 2002 the states have had to close a cumulative budget gap of more than $235 billion (NCSL, 2004:1). Higher education, a recipient of state funding for research and research infrastructure, has been especially hard hit, resulting in tuition increases in several states.

The states support R&D through various mechanisms, including direct appropriations to universities, R&D tax credits, the establishment of endowment funds, and the formation of nonprofit corporations. Although there is no complete database of state expenditures for health research, some studies of spending have been conducted by national organizations of both state support of health research or biotechnology and state use of tobacco settlement funds for research. Specific examples, such as Ohio's Center for Stem Cell and Regenerative Medicine and the North Carolina Biotechnology Center, provide illustrations of the types of initiatives more likely to be undertaken and funded by states.

Most states also have economic development programs interested in funding medical research and biotechnology, with money that would not otherwise be spent on medical research (Battelle/SSTI, 2004). But states, like industry, are generally most interested in research that will have immediate commercial appli-

---

[8]See www.nationalhealthcouncil.org/pubs/research_00.htm.

BOX 2-2
The Juvenile Diabetes Research Foundation International

JDRF is the leading charitable funder and advocate of type 1 diabetes research worldwide. To date, JDRF has awarded more than $680 million for diabetes research. The foundation seeks to find a cure for diabetes and its complications by supporting multidisciplinary programs that bring together diabetes researchers from numerous institutions, private and public, and from diverse disciplines.

JDRF also seeks to leverage its research impact by partnering with and stimulating increased research spending on the part of public and private medical organizations and other entities throughout the world. In FY 2003, JDRF provided $80.0 million, funding 500 centers, grants, and fellowships in 19 countries. Thirty-eight percent of its funding is spent outside the United States, often in partnerships with other governments. JDRF funding and leadership have been associated with most major scientific breakthroughs in type 1 diabetes research to date.

In its collaborations with the federal government, JDRF has participated in numerous partnerships with NIH that have added value on both sides of the table, with NIH providing most of the funding and generally operating the programs. JDRF works to maximize the impact of its funding by complementing, not duplicating, NIH efforts. This year begins the second five-year term of earmarked money—$150.0 million per year for five years over and above the normal NIH appropriation for type 1 diabetes—which gives JDRF leverage in working with the agency on how the money is spent. One specific partnership with NIH, TrialNet, involves a consortium approach using cooperative agreements to conduct clinical trials for type 1 diabetes related to new onset, prevention of the disease, or amelioration of further damage. For this project, JDRF is providing funding to include four international sites in the consortium, an example of how foundation partnering can make a significant difference.

Another JDRF partnership involves DOD, the National Aeronautics and Space

cations, as this helps to build the state's biotechnology industry and thus increase the number of jobs. States also are investing in the biomedical R&D capacity of their universities and other research institutions to enable them to compete more effectively for support from federal agencies—especially NIH—and industry and foundations. Most state economic development funds aim to leverage multiple federal dollars for each state dollar, not the other way around.

A few states, such as California and New Jersey, have peer reviewed research grant programs, but these are small relative to federal programs, and they concentrate on leveraging federal funds by supporting exploratory research projects and new investigators to help state medical researchers win R01 (traditional individual investigator-initiated) grants from NIH.

State revenues can be affected by the ups and downs of the business cycle, because they must balance their budgets each year. This makes it more difficult

Administration, and NIH working together to develop technologies for metabolic monitoring through the Technologies for Metabolic Monitoring and Julia Weaver Fund Research Program, managed by the U.S. Army Medical Research and Materiel Command. This year JDRF will spend about $3.5 million to fund this research, which is targeted at developing a means to understand, predict, and closely monitor metabolic products, with an emphasis on monitoring blood glucose levels. The scientific interests of DOD and JDRF come together in this effort, with DOD seeking a remote, noninvasive way to detect metabolic arrangements, while JDRF would like to have a glucose monitor. JDRF also partners with the Defense Advanced Research Projects Agency, which has a mutual interest in research on tissue regeneration and repair.

JDRF plays an important and unique role in setting the global direction of diabetes research resources to ensure that they are used as effectively as possible. JDRF's many international partnerships fund specific aspects of type 1 diabetes, while also bringing to the table the resources of the governments of each country involved, including their research councils. The international partnerships allow for effective leveraging of resources, as occurred, for example, when JDRF partnered with the Swedish Medical Research Council and the Knut & Alice Wallennberg Foundation to support a five-year program involving research networks in type 1 diabetes. Another project involves the Swedish Research Council, the Swedish Diabetes Association, and JDRF working together to support stem cell research.

JDRF's experience with these kinds of partnerships, coupled with its desire to promote stem cell research beyond the NIH guidelines, led to early talks with the Medical Research Council of the United Kingdom. In January 2002, the Council sponsored the formation of the International Stem Cell Forum. Currently, the Forum consists of 18 international funders of research with an interest in working together to further stem cell research. JDRF is the only nongovernment partner in this collaboration, one that provides an example of what can be accomplished through partnerships that provide not only money, but also scientific interest.

for them to provide long-term support of research programs. Nevertheless, states do fund medical research and likely would be interested in partnering with federal programs such as CDMRP on projects of mutual interest. As mentioned previously, some states have established programs to support biomedical research, or all areas of research, with dedicated funding from the tobacco settlement or other sources of regular revenues, such as state tobacco taxes.

State Support for Health Research and Development

In 1998, Battelle and the State Science and Technology Institute (SSTI) conducted a survey of state funding of R&D for NSF. The study found that states spent $3.0 billion on R&D and R&D plants in FY 1995—$2.7 billion from their own sources and the rest from federal programs, industry, and foundations

(Battelle/SSTI, 1998). The states, which were asked to report spending by functional category and by scientific field, identified $278.0 million as health R&D, but $1.0 billion as biological, medical, and psychological research. Evidently, some states included funding of state university research in a separate category called "science and technology base."

In 2001, McGeary and Smith conducted a study of state funding of health research for the Lasker Foundation, finding that data sources were scattered and incomplete (McGeary and Smith, 2001). But by extrapolating the 1995 survey data and adding tobacco settlement funding spent on research as well as other state programs established since 1995, the authors estimated that states were spending about $2.0 billion in 2001 on health research. Since 2001 tobacco settlement revenues have increased, but the fiscal crisis in many states has caused them to shift the revenue from programs to debt reduction. Much health research funding occurs through state colleges and universities and their medical centers, but this funding is probably already highly leveraged through cost sharing on federal grants and contracts.

According to a 2004 survey of state bioscience initiatives conducted for the Biotechnology Industry Organization, 40 states are investing in the development of bioscience and technology as a means of economic development and job creation (Battelle/SSTI, 2004:28). In general, the strategies are to encourage biotechnology firms to locate in the states, enhance the biomedical research capacity of state universities and other research institutions, foster greater industry-university interaction, build modern facilities with wet-lab space and specialized equipment to attract new firms, and create publicly supported commercialization, seed, and venture capital funds that can invest in bioscience-related companies (see Box 2-3 for an example).

Some states use state funds to support research projects that can leverage funding from merit-based federal science programs that need nonfederal investment in facilities or equipment to be competitive or that require nonfederal cost sharing. Firms can sometimes be induced to fund R&D in an area of mutual interest if the state will share the costs, and local foundations sometimes will contribute funds if they are interested in economic development as a means of expanding economic opportunities. Currently, 23 states have programs of biomedical research grants or centers of excellence, or both; 33 provide funding for biomedical research facilities; 9 have biomedical faculty development programs; 32 have university-related research parks (12 of them specifically for biotechnology enterprises); 33 offer R&D tax credits; and 17 have university-industry matching grant programs (Battelle/SSTI, 2004: Table 6).

State Expenditures of Tobacco Settlement Revenue

Many states planned on using funds from the 1998 Tobacco Master Settlement, when it was signed, for research purposes, particularly those addressing

BOX 2-3
Example of State-Funded Biotechnology Development: North Carolina Biotechnology Center

In 1981, North Carolina's General Assembly established the North Carolina Biotechnology Center (NCBC) as a private, nonprofit (close nonprofit) corporation that would provide economic benefit to the state through supporting biotechnology R&D and commercialization. NCBC works in partnership with the North Carolina Department of Commerce, the North Carolina Biosciences Organization, the Council for Entrepreneurial Development, the University of North Carolina system, the Community College system, private universities, the Small Business and Technology Development Center, Golden LEAF (tobacco settlement fund program), Chambers of Commerce, and many other groups. For the past 15 years, NCBC has received annually an average of $7.0 million from the state through bipartisan legislative support (NCBC, 1999). This funding comes mainly from state appropriations, but also from federal and private sector funds. The pharmaceutical partners helped build the center where NCBC is based. NCBC's total annual budget is approximately $10.0 million, which is spent on research, workforce development and education programs, venture capital investment, and other activities (Alexandre, 2004). The amount spent on research depends on how much is allocated within the given year. For 2004, grant programs total approximately $3 to $4 million and are invested into various research programs. NCBC funds mostly transitional and applied research, rather than basic research, and has three core programs: Science and Technology Development, Business and Technology Development, and Education and Training. Other state-funded initiatives include the North Carolina Genomics and Bioinformatics Consortium, which promotes genomics, proteomics, and bioinformatics.

tobacco-related illnesses. According to the report of the National Governors Association's Center for Best Practices on tobacco settlement spending, 17 states (of the 46 that reported) allocated some portion of funding specifically to biomedical and health research, which includes research projects on cancer and tobacco-related diseases (NGA, 2001:3).

Since 2001, there has been a steady decline in the percentage of tobacco settlement funds used by states for health (this category includes medical research but not capital expenditures for research facilities). In 2003, 24 percent of the funding went to health (most of the funding went for deficit reduction), but only 17 percent is estimated for 2004. The states allocated about 36 percent of tobacco settlement funds to reduce budget shortfalls and are expected to allocate about 54 percent in 2004 (U.S. GAO, 2004). Thirteen states allocated tobacco settlement funds for health research in 2003—Arkansas, Florida, Georgia, Illinois, Louisiana, Maryland, Michigan, Nebraska, New Mexico, Ohio (see Box 2-4), Pennsylvania,

BOX 2-4
Example of State-Funded Medical Research: Ohio's Third Frontier Project

In 2003, Ohio Governor Bob Taft awarded a capital grant (through the state's Wright Centers of Innovation Program) for $10.8 million to help build the Center for Stem Cell and Regenerative Medicine in Cleveland and another $8.6 million to finance research there. The center is a research collaboration among Case Western Reserve University, Cleveland Clinic, University Hospitals of Cleveland, Ohio State University, and seven industry partners (including Cleveland-based Athersys, Inc.). Funding for the center's research comes from Ohio's Biomedical Research and Technology Transfer Fund, which was created by the state's share of tobacco settlement. The center is part of Ohio's Third Frontier Project, a state initiative formed to create high-technology jobs by supporting research.

Texas, and Utah. The percentages each state allocated for health research ranged from 0.2 percent in Texas to 28.7 percent in Maryland. The total, $278.9 million, was 2.3 percent of the $12.2 billion received by the states from the tobacco settlement in 2003.

SUMMARY

Several sources of nonfederal funding for medical R&D exist in the United States. The largest contributor is private industry, with the pharmaceutical industry alone providing over $32.0 billion in 2003. Most of the industrial investment is at the development end of the R&D spectrum; thus, interest in CDMRP programs would likely be focused primarily on ideas or projects that are ready for scale-up and production. Likewise, U.S. venture capital markets are more likely to seek opportunities where the likelihood of near-term payoff is greater. Although academia provides some funds and in-kind support for research, public universities in particular have been struggling with budget reductions caused by state fiscal constraints.

Philanthropic organizations, foundations, and public charities also make an important, but smaller, contribution to health research of approximately $1.0 billion annually. These groups tend to find ways to leverage the much larger federal and industrial investment and frequently support focused areas of research specific to one disease or set of disorders. Finally, states provide roughly $2.0 billion annually in support of bioscience-related R&D activities. Much of this investment is focused on employment and economic development.

REFERENCES

AAFRC (American Association of Fundraising Counsel). 2004. Americans Give $241 Billion to Charity in 2003 [press release]. [On-line.] Available: aafrc.org/press_releases/trustreleases/americansgive.html [accessed July 18, 2004].

Alexandre LM. 2004. Presentation by President and CEO of the North Carolina Biotechnology Center at workshop held by the Committee on Alternative Funding Strategies for DOD's Peer Reviewed Medical Research Programs. National Academies, Washington, DC, April 27.

AUTM (Association of University Technology Managers). 2002. *AUTM Licensing Survey: FY 2002: A Survey Summary of Technology Licensing (and Related) Performance for U.S. and Canadian Academic and Nonprofit Institutions, and Patent Management and Investment Firms.* Northbrook, IL: AUTM [On-line.] Available: www.autm.net/index_ie.html [accessed July 18, 2004].

Battelle/SSTI (Science and Technology Institute). 1998. *Survey of State Research and Development Expenditures, Fiscal Year 1995.* Westerville, OH: Science and Technology Institute.

Battelle/SSTI. 2004. *Laboratories of Innovation: State Bioscience Initiatives 2004.* Prepared for BIO—Biotechnology Industry Organization, Washington, D.C. [On-line.] Available: www.bio.org/speeches/pubs/battelle2004.pdf [accessed June 14, 2004].

Bond EC, Peck MG, Scott M. 1999. *The Future of Philanthropic Support for Medical/Health Research.* [On-line.] Available: www.aaas.org/spp/dspp/cstc/fundscience/papers/bond.htm.

Foundation Center. 2004. *Foundation Giving Trends, 2004.* New York, NY: The Foundation Center. [Summary on-line.] Available: www.foundationcenter.org/research/trends_analy-sis/pdf/04fgthiltes.pdf [accessed July 18, 2004].

Lichtman MA, Hunter MD, Liders GJ. 2004. "Intellectual Property—The Dispute between Research Institutions and Voluntary Health Agencies." *Nature Biotechnology*, 22(4):385-386.

McGeary M, Smith PM. 2001. *State Support for Medical Research: Report on State Support for Health Research for Funding First.* Washington, DC: McGeary and Smith, October 26. [On-line.] Available: www.laskerfoundation.com/ffpages/reports/m1.htm [accessed July 18, 2004].

McNichol E, Harris M. 2004. *Many States Cut Budgets as Fiscal Squeeze Continues.* Washington, DC: Center on Budget and Policy Priorities, April 26. [On-line.] Available: www.cbpp.org/pubs/sfp.htm [accessed July 18, 2004].

NCBC (North Carolina Biotechnology Center). 1999. *North Carolina Biotechnology Center: A Progress Report 1984-1999.* [On-line.] Available: www.ncbiotech.org/pdffiles/progress.pdf [accessed July 20, 2004].

NCSL (National Conference of State Legislatures). 2004. *State Budge & Tax Actions 2004: Preliminary Report.* [On-line.] Available: www.ncsl.org/programs/fiscal/presbta04.htm#note4 [accessed July 12, 2004].

NGA (National Governors Association). 2001. 2001 State Tobacco Settlement Spending Initiatives (Issue Brief). Washington, DC: NGA Center for Best Practices. [On-line.] Available: www.nga.org/cda/files/IB200104111SPENDING.pdf [accessed July 18, 2004].

NIH (National Institutes of Health). 2004a. *Federal Obligations for Health R&D, by Source or Performer, Fiscal Years 1985-2001.* [On-line]. Available: grants.nih.gov/grants/award/research/sourfund.htm [accessed May 20, 2004].

NIH. 2004b. *Federal Agencies Health R&D by Performer.* [On-line]. Available: grants.nih.gov/grants/award/research/performr.htm [accessed June 29, 2004].

NSF (National Science Foundation). 2002. Memorandum, Christine C. Boesz, Inspector General, NSF, to Warren Washington, Chair, National Science Board, and Rita R. Colwell, Director, NSF, "Management Challenges for NSF in 2003." Arlington, VA: NSF, December 23.

NSF. 2003a. *Research and Development in Industry: 2000.* NSF 03-318. Arlington, VA: NSF. [On-line.] Available: www.nsf.gov/sbe/srs/nsf03318/start.htm [accessed July 18, 2004].

NSF. 2003b. *Academic Research and Development Expenditures: Fiscal Year 2001*. NSF 03-316. Arlington, VA: NSF. [On-line.] Available: www.nsf.gov/sbe/srs/nsf03316/start.htm [accessed July 18, 2004].

NSF. 2004a. *Science and Engineering Indicators 2004*. Two volumes: volume 1, NSB 04-1; volume 2, NSB 04-1A. Arlington, VA: National Science Board, NSF. [On-line.] Available: www.nsf.gov/sbe/srs/seind04/start.htm [accessed July 18, 2004].

NSF. 2004b. *U.S. Academic R&D Continues to Grow as More Universities and Colleges Expand Their R&D Activities* (NSF InfoBrief). NSF 04-319. Arlington, VA: NSF. [On-line.] Available: www.nsf.gov/sbe/srs/infbrief/nsf04319/start.htm [accessed July 18, 2004].

NVCA (National Venture Capital Association). 2004a. *What Is Venture Capital?* [Online.] Available: www.nvca.org/def.html [accessed July 12, 2004].

NVCA. 2004b. Venture Capital Stays the Course in Q1 2004 with $4.6 billion Invested (Press Release). [Online.] Available: www.nvca.org/pdf/Q104MTReleaseEmbargoFINAL.pdf [accessed July 12, 2004].

PhRMA (Pharmaceutical Research and Manufacturers of America). 1997. *New Medicines in Development for Cancer: 1997 Survey*. Washington, DC: PhRMA.

PhRMA. 2003. *Medicines in Development for Cancer: 2003 Survey*. Washington, DC: PhRMA, May. [On-line.] Available: www.phrma.org/newmedicines/resources/2003-05-12.109.pdf [accessed May 20, 2004].

PhRMA. 2004. *Pharmaceutical Industry Profile 2004*. Washington, DC: PhRMA. [On-line.] Available: www.phrma.org/publications/publications//2004-03-31.937.pdf [accessed May 20, 2004].

R!A (Research!America). 2003. *2001 Investment in U.S. Health Research* [Issue Paper]. Alexandria, VA: R!A. Data supplied by Stacie Propst, Ph.D.

R!A. 2004. *2002 Investment in U.S. Health Research* [Issue Paper]. Alexandria, VA: R!A. [On-line.] Available: www.researchamerica.org/publications/appropriations/healthdollar2002.pdf [accessed July 18 2004].

U.S. GAO (U.S. General Accounting Office). 2004. *Tobacco Settlement: States' Allocations of Fiscal Year 2003 and Expected Fiscal Year 2004 Payments*. GAO-04-518. Washington, DC: GAO. [On-line.] Available: www.gao.gov/new.items/d04518.pdf [accessed July 18, 2004].

3

Examples of Leveraging Nonfederal Dollars for Research

Research funding approaches taken by federal agencies offer many examples of how nonfederal resources have been mobilized in support of federal research and development (R&D) programs. A number of examples of federal R&D programs that involve nonfederal funding are briefly described in Appendix A (many more exist that the committee could not document in the short time it had to gather information). Although these initiatives exhibit a wide variety of characteristics, most can be usefully grouped along two dimensions:

1. The nonfederal resources in a federal R&D program may be required or they may be provided voluntarily.
2. The responsibility for securing the nonfederal resources may fall to the applicant and his or her institution or to the federal funding agency.

These two dimensions provide a typology (see Table 3-1).

It is noted that most cases cluster in the upper left-hand and lower right-hand corners of this quadrant. This is because resources from industry, philanthropy, and other sources are not usually reported to federal agencies unless such reporting is required for matching purposes and because in some cases federal agencies cannot require the provision of funds from the private sector or from state and local government to be a condition of making an award.

This chapter provides some examples of each category of nonfederal support for federal research projects, with a number of additional examples described briefly in Appendix A (many more exist that the committee could not document in the short time it had to gather information).

TABLE 3-1 Typology of Federal/Nonfederal Funding Arrangements

	Required	Voluntary
Awardee Level	I. Cost Sharing or Matching Required of Awardees	II. Voluntary Cost Sharing by Awardees
Agency Level	III. Nonfederal Funding Secured by Federal Agency	IV. Nonfederal Funding Volunteered to Federal Agency

COST SHARING OR MATCHING REQUIRED OF AWARDEES

In federal parlance, cost sharing usually is defined as an arrangement in which a portion of a federal project's or program's costs are not borne by the federal government. Matching of funds is often considered to be a special case of cost sharing in which the federal government matches private or state funding for a program dollar for dollar (Feller, 1997). Matching also usually implies the provision of cash rather than in-kind contributions. However, these terms are not used consistently, even within federal policy documents. For example, in the Office of Management and Budget's (OMB's) Circular A-110, "Uniform Administrative Requirements for Grants and Agreements with Institutes of Higher Education and Other Non-Profit Organizations," cost sharing and matching are treated as interchangeable terms. In this report, cost sharing will be used as the general term for all costs contributed to a research project by an awardee institution from sources other than the federal award. Matching is the special case of cost sharing in which the awardee institution must match federal funding dollar for dollar, either in cash or through in-kind contributions, or a combination of both.

The amount of cost sharing may be a specific percentage of the total funding, a minimum or maximum percentage of the total funding, or it can be open ended. Industry or another nonfederal organization might be the source of the cost sharing.

Cost sharing may be a condition of eligibility to apply for funds or it may be a criterion of proposal review, as many federal agencies require the applicant organization to pay part of the cost of an R&D project. As an eligibility condition, the applicant must show in the proposed budget where the required percentage of cost sharing is applied and must provide letters of commitment from the sources of cost sharing. In these cases, cost sharing is usually a fixed percentage or a minimum percentage. In other cases, cost sharing is encouraged rather than required, with one of the review criteria being the extent of university or industry commitment, either monetary or in kind (see, for example, U.S. Army Research Office, 2003). Matching award amounts can be increased during review, or a ceiling may be imposed on the amount of matching funds that can be provided in order to prevent a bidding war among applicants.

Cost Sharing in Selected Federal Programs

The appropriations laws providing funds to the National Science Foundation (NSF) require the recipients of grants and contracts to share in the costs of projects that are not specifically solicited by NSF. In accordance with this statutory requirement, NSF requires projects initiated by investigators to be cost shared at a level equal to 1 percent of the total cost (NSF, 2002a). Grantee institutions may either cost share a minimum of 1 percent on each project or cost share a minimum of 1 percent on the aggregate total cost for all projects (that is, share a greater percentage on some projects and not share at all on other projects). Although the 1 percent cost share is not included in the proposal budget, it must be accounted for in the awardee's records and is subject to audit.

At one time, the National Institutes of Health (NIH) required cost sharing on all grants, but this provision has been dropped in most cases (although there might be cost-sharing requirements for salaries funded through awards). The National Aeronautics and Space Administration (NASA) does not require cost sharing on research grants and cooperative agreements with universities and other nonprofit institutions, because "their activities generally do not produce benefits that can be measured as having significance apart from the benefit intrinsic in conducting research for NASA" (NASA, n.d.). NASA accepts voluntary cost sharing, but it is not supposed to be a factor in the decision to make an award. Cost sharing is not generally required or considered in the evaluation and selection process for grants and cooperative agreements awarded by the Office of Science at the Department of Energy (DOE), although it may be required in certain awards, for example, those for research equipment.[1]

CDMRP has a cost-sharing requirement, which is deemed to be met when recipients provide the equipment needed to support proposed research. In the case of training grants, the award covers only the trainee's stipend. Mentoring time and other activities involved in the training are in effect in-kind donations provided by the Principal Investigator and his or her institution. This cost sharing is not included in the budget or accounted for by the awardee institution, which reduces the administrative burden on both the grantee and CDMRP.[2] It is expected, however, that grantee institutions will share 50 percent of the cost of equipment purchased for a research proposal when individual equipment costs are equal to or exceed $5,000.

---

[1] 10 CFR Part 605, Office of Energy Research Financial Assistance Program, Section 605.13, Cost Sharing. See www.er.doe.gov/production/grants/605.html [accessed May 18, 2004].

[2] If the approved project involves the purchase of equipment costing $5,000 or more, however, the institution must share half the cost.

NSF Engineering Research Centers and Other NSF Programs

The NSF Engineering Research Centers (ERCs) Program was created in 1985 to develop a government-industry-university partnership that would strengthen the competitive position of U.S. firms in world trade. ERCs are university based, with 80 percent of their funding coming from NSF and 20 percent from industry, states, and other sources. Cost sharing is employed as a means of ensuring that the research and other activities of an ERC are considered important and relevant enough to justify investment by the center's industrial members and to give industry a stake in the performance of the center. Cost sharing also is justified by the general principle that recipients should pay a portion of the costs when they stand to benefit from the project.

According to current NSF policy, cost sharing can be used only as an eligibility requirement, not as a factor in the review process (NSF, 2002b). Additional voluntary cost sharing also is not considered in the peer review process; it is not included in the materials that are provided to peer reviewers.

An ERC develops partnerships with member firms and other practitioner organizations (e.g., hospitals and state and local government agencies) to facilitate an exchange of information, provide mentors for students, speed technology transfer, and identify sources of financial support. Member organizations serve on the ERC's Industrial/Practitioner Advisory Board and are expected to provide access to industrial facilities and personnel for ERC faculty and students, knowledge of industrial practice, and awareness of the areas that are in need of future technological innovation.

Member organizations pay cash membership fees, generally on a sliding-fee scale according to the size of the firm. Members also may provide the center in-kind and sponsored project support or provide support directly to ERC faculty for sponsored projects that contribute directly to the center's strategic plan. Some centers also receive cash and in-kind donations from nonmember organizations. Annual funding for centers ranges from \$3.1 million to \$19.4 million. NSF's contribution ranges from \$1.0 million to \$3.0 million per year, averaging \$2.5 million per year.

Cost sharing at a level equal to 20 percent or more of the total amount requested from NSF must be shown and justified in the proposal budget. An awardee's contribution to cost sharing is limited to items that, if charged to the project, would be allowable under applicable cost principles contained in OMB's Circular A-110. Contributions may be cash or in kind, but they must be from a nonfederal source. In addition, contributions counted as cost sharing toward projects of another federal agency may not be counted toward meeting the cost-sharing requirement of an ERC award.

Other NSF programs require cost sharing. They include center programs, such as Science and Technology Centers (30 percent), Materials Research Science and Engineering Centers (10 percent), Nanoscale Research and Engineering

Centers (10 percent), and Industry/University Cooperative Research Centers (of variable percentages). They also include instrumentation awards, such as Chemistry Research Instrumentation and Facilities grants for departmental multi-user instruments (50 percent of costs over the first $100,000).[3]

National Cancer Institute Academic Public-Private Partnerships

Recently, the National Cancer Institute (NCI) launched the Academic Public-Private Partnership Program (AP4), a new initiative aimed at combining the basic research skills within academic institutions, the scientific expertise of industry, the interests of disease-oriented charities and nonprofit groups, and the administrative support, resources, and discovery and development expertise of NCI. The purpose of establishing academic-public-private partnerships is to conduct novel cancer therapeutic, prevention, diagnostic, and imaging research to hasten the translation of research findings into clinical trials. The research will take place at academic centers with the advice and support of their industrial, nonprofit, and state government partners.

The program is modeled after NSF's Industry/University Cooperative Research Center Program, in which NSF's share of the funding declines over time and the center is eventually fully supported by its nonfederal partners. NCI currently is issuing 1-year planning grants, but NCI intends to provide a 10-year grant of $450,000 per year in direct costs to university-based centers, with industry, nonprofit, and/or state and local government partners contributing at least $300,000 per year. The NCI contribution would drop to $337,500 in year 4, $225,000 in year 5, and between $100,000 and $200,000 in years 6 through 10.[4] The 10-year grant is not renewable.

National Institute of Allergy and Infectious Diseases Challenge Grants

In this program, the National Institute of Allergy and Infectious Diseases (NIAID) matches funding from companies for product development that has commercial potential. The program was launched in fiscal year (FY) 2000 by a special appropriation of $20 million.

The first solicitation, in FY 2000, resulted in challenge grants totaling $18 million to eight companies for the development of drugs and vaccines against major infectious diseases, such as malaria, tuberculosis (TB), influenza, and

---

[3]Program Solicitation NSF 03-563, "Chemistry Research Instrumentation and Facilities: Departmental Multi-User Instrumentation," July 3, 2004.

[4]If the partnership can contribute at least $450,000 in nonfederal funding, NCI will provide $600,000 in years 1-3, $450,000 in year 4, $300,000 in year 3, and $100,000 to $200,000 in years 6 through 10.

emerging and resistant infections.[5] One project resulted in first new vaccine for TB to enter human clinical trials in more than 60 years.

NIAID has issued another challenge grant solicitation looking for candidate products that are ready for further development. It calls for collaborative partnerships between government and the private sector to further develop already-identified products against NIAID Category A, B, and C high-priority pathogens and all stages of product development against Severe Acute Respiratory Syndrome (SARS), including vaccines, adjuvants, therapeutics, diagnostics, and research resources.[6]

Cost Sharing by Universities and Other Recipient Research Institutions

Grantee institutions already share costs to the extent that indirect cost recovery does not cover the full expenses of research.[7] OMB caps administrative costs, and some federal R&D programs do not pay the full indirect cost rate. Most major research universities have administrative costs that exceed the cap, and administrative costs have been steadily increasing because of new and expanded federal regulations, such as the Health Insurance Portability and Accountability Act (HIPAA); the USA Patriot Act and its requisite control of Select Biological Agents; environmental health and safety rules; and policies for the protection of human subjects in research (COGR, 2003; Goldman and Williams, 2000). State universities receive lower indirect cost recovery rates than do private universities, with the difference essentially becoming a state subsidy of federally funded research. According to an NSF survey, universities fund about 20 percent of the R&D conducted in their facilities, of which approximately half comes from indirect cost recovery (NSF, 2004). The other half comes from tuition, gifts and bequests, and endowments, much of which is already counted as cost sharing on federal awards.

VOLUNTARY COST SHARING BY AWARDEES

Cost sharing is usually one of the review criteria for a proposal rather than a condition of application eligibility in this small category. Some agencies, such as NSF, have stopped allowing open-ended cost sharing because of undesirable effects, which include the offering of cost sharing as a competitive tactic by

[5]RFA-AI-00-010, "Challenge Grants: Joint Ventures in Biomedicine and Biotechnology," February 10, 2000.

[6]RFA-AI-03-016, "Challenge Grants: Biodefense and SARS Product Development," September 22, 2003.

[7]According to a recent RAND study, universities recover between 70 percent and 90 percent of their overhead costs in conducting federally funded research (Goldman and Williams, 2000).

applicants, the appearance that a successful applicant "bought" the award, the unequal capacities of applicant institutions to provide cost sharing, the insertion of financial considerations into the peer review process, reduced ability to fund technically excellent proposals with low cost sharing, and the entrepreneurial use of cost sharing by program managers to stretch program funding to fund more grants (Feller, 1997). In 1999, NSF adopted a new cost-sharing policy in which the amount of cost sharing is specified and is treated as an eligibility criterion rather than a review criterion (NSF, 1999).

U.S. Army Collaborative Technology Alliances

In 2001, the Army Research Laboratory (ARL) awarded five cooperative agreements for Collaborative Technology Alliances in the areas of advanced sensors, power and energy, advanced decision architecture, communications and networks, and robotics.[8] These five-year awards of $35 million each included an option of $20 million in additional funding for three more years.

Each alliance is a consortium whose members have signed Articles of Collaboration. Each consortium has a lead company and a dozen or more other partners, divided between companies and universities. All are represented on a consortium management committee, along with a representative of ARL. According to the program announcement, the intent was:

> to create a critical mass of private sector and government scientists and engineers focused on solving the Army's technology challenges, as well as supporting and stimulating dual-use applications of this research and technology to benefit commercial use.[9]

The program announcement also states that:

> Cost sharing is not required . . . however, it is strongly encouraged. During the evaluation of proposals, cost sharing will be evaluated as it relates to the evaluation factors set forth in the Program Announcement, based on the degree to which the proposed cost sharing enhances the proposal to result in added benefits to the program.

NONFEDERAL FUNDING SECURED BY FEDERAL AGENCIES

Technically, federal agencies cannot require nonfederal entities, such as companies and states, to provide funding for federal research programs. However, one type of arrangement that comes close includes cases in which an agency and

---

[8]See www.arl.army.mil.alliances/ [accessed May 17, 2004].

[9]U.S. Army Research Laboratory, Program Announcement/Solicitation, "Collaborative Technology Alliances," August 11, 2000. At www.arl.mil/alliances/final.doc [accessed May 17, 2004].

an entity in another sector agree to a long-term funding arrangement that each side is committed to fund each year. Another arrangement includes awards that contain a provision to recoup federal costs stemming from the successful commercialization of a technology produced by federally funded R&D, with the recouped costs to be cycled back into the program for future research. An example of each kind of arrangement follows.

Health Effects Institute

The Health Effects Institute (HEI) is an independent nonprofit corporation chartered in 1980 to provide high-quality, impartial, and relevant scientific research on the health effects of pollutants from motor vehicles and other environmental sources. It is supported by the U.S. Environmental Protection Agency (EPA) and 27 automobile companies, which match the EPA contribution through a series of five-year agreements. Each company contributes in proportion to its North American sales.

HEI has funded more than 170 studies and has published more than 100 research reports and several special reports that have included important research findings on the health effects of a variety of pollutants, including carbon monoxide, methanol and aldehydes, nitrogen oxides, diesel exhaust, ozone, and most recently, particulate air pollution. HEI also has been called on periodically to produce special reports that review an entire area of scientific literature on topics such as the health effects of asbestos, diesel exhaust, and oxygenates in fuel.

To accomplish its mission, HEI:

- identifies the highest priority areas for health effects research;
- funds and oversees the conduct of high-quality research in these priority areas;
- provides intensive, independent review of HEI-supported and related research;
- integrates HEI's research results with those of other institutions into coherent, broader evaluations of health effects; and
- communicates the results of HEI research and analyses to public and private decisionmakers.

HEI is governed by a Board of Directors that is chaired by Richard Celeste, ex-governor of Ohio, and includes public figures in science and policy. The institute's scientific work is overseen by two independent scientific committees. The Health Research Committee works with the institute's scientific staff to develop and manage HEI's research program, while the Health Review Committee, which has no role in selecting or overseeing studies, works with the institute's scientific staff to evaluate and interpret the results of HEI studies and related research.

A third committee, the Special Committee on Emerging Technologies, advises HEI on new technologies and fuels and their potential health and environmental impact. Its membership was selected to provide a broad range of technical expertise from government, industry, public interest, and academic organizations.

HEI's priorities for research and special reviews are guided by the five-year HEI Strategic Plan, which is reviewed and updated annually after consultations with HEI sponsors and other interested parties.

This strategy of creating a jointly funded subsidiary was probably first employed in the establishment of SEMATECH in 1987. SEMATECH was funded with $100 million per year from the federal government, matched by a total of $100 million per year from nearly all the large semiconductor companies in the United States.

Clean Coal Power Initiative

The Clean Coal Power Initiative of DOE is a $2 billion, 10-year program of investment in joint government-industry projects to develop innovative technologies for coal-fired power plants. For this initiative, which is primarily a cost-sharing program, industrial sponsors must match the federal funding share by contributing at least half of the total amount of funds. There also is a requirement for repayment from commercially successful technologies that result from the effort, which will be used to fund additional clean coal research.

According to DOE's announcement of funding opportunity for the second round of funding ($280 million), DOE is inviting proposals that will be competitively reviewed and funded by cooperative agreements with "at least 50% cost sharing" (DOE, 2004). In 2003, DOE announced the selection of eight projects receiving $316 million in federal funds matched by more than $1 billion in private funds (there were 36 proposals submitted with more than $5 billion in matching funds).

Proposals must include information on the awardee's repayment plan that meets the following conditions:

> DOE expects repayment plans to be realistic and to provide a reasonable plan for achieving 100% repayment of DOE's actual contribution to the project. Repayment may come from various revenue streams including, but not limited to, those from the demonstration project itself, royalties from sales and licensing of the technology in the United States and abroad, and/or any other source of funds the applicant chooses to propose. (DOE, 2004)

Some private sector funders also seek recoupment. Genentech, for example, is collaborating with Accelerate Brain Cancer Cure (ABC^2), a nonprofit foundation, on the development of new therapies for patients with brain cancer, in an arrangement in which the two organizations share expenses. Genentech uses the clinical network created by ABC^2, and ABC^2 shares royalties from any treatments that are approved for use.[10] In another example, grants from the American Institute for Cancer Research (AICR) have a provision that allows AICR to share in any royalty income that might result from a patentable invention made in the course of research supported in whole or in part by its funds.[11]

NONFEDERAL FUNDING VOLUNTEERED TO FEDERAL AGENCIES

Some federal agencies have the authority to accept contributions designated for specific purposes. NIH institutes, for example, receive a number of gifts and bequests each year for ongoing research on a particular disease or for a designated program. Increasingly, an agency and a nonfederal entity or entities, such as a company, foundation, or voluntary health agency (VHA), agree to support a new research initiative jointly.

Several arrangements are possible, including the following: (1) some or all of the collaborators agree to pool their funds for the initiative; (2) the collaborators contribute in complementary ways, for example, each agreeing to fund a particular part of the whole initiative; (3) a nonfederal entity agrees to supplement a federal award; (4) a nonfederal entity piggybacks on a federal program by funding projects that receive high peer review ratings but that lack agency funds for support; or (5) nonfederal partners contribute in other ways, such as referring patients or encouraging members to provide biological samples for a federally funded project. Examples of each of these arrangements follow.

Pooling of Federal and Nonfederal Funds

NIH provides the best example of a case in which private funds have been added to federal funds for a program of research grants. Private organizations that fund medical research are aware that NIH is authorized by the Public Health Service Act to receive conditional gifts, or contributions, for specific purposes.[12] The Office of the General Counsel of the Department of Health and Human Services has determined, however, that although this authority provides a mechanism to NIH for accepting funds from outside sources, NIH employees may not actively solicit funds to augment appropriated funds.[13] NIH instead has begun working through the Foundation for the National Institutes of Health (FNIH) to

---

[10] See the press announcement of the ABC^2-Genentech collaboration at www.abc2.org/news_02252002.htm.

[11] See AICR's patent policy at www.aicr.org/research/patents.lasso.

[12] Sections 231 and 405(b)(1)(H) of the Public Health Service Act, as amended (42 U.S.C. §§238,284(b)(1)(H).

[13] NIH Policy Manual, Chapter 1135, "Gifts Administration," Part E8, "Solicitation Prohibited." See www.od.nih.gov/oma/manualchapters/management/1135/main.html.

organize research collaborations, raise funds from private sources such as companies and foundations, and transfer the money to NIH.

FNIH is a nonprofit charitable organization founded to support NIH in its mission. It is tax exempt under section 501(c)(3) of the Internal Revenue Code, and gifts to FNIH are tax deductible. Moreover, its congressional charter makes it the only acceptable financial intermediary for the third-party donation of funds to NIH.[14] FNIH has been the mechanism for pooling private funds with NIH funds for several initiatives, including the Mouse Sequencing Consortium, the Multilateral Initiative on Malaria, Overcoming Barriers to Early Phase Clinical Trials, and the Osteoarthritis Initiative Public-Private Consortium (described below). Several more, modeled on the Osteoarthritis Initiative, are in development, including the National Institute on Aging's (NIA's) Alzheimer's Disease Neuroimaging Initiative and NCI's Image Database Resources Initiative of the National Cancer Institute. Each involves contributions from companies and, in some cases, foundations and VHAs that are made to a program of NIH-reviewed and NIH-funded grants.

The Centers for Disease Control and Prevention (CDC) has a similar arrangement with the CDC Foundation, an independent nonprofit organization established in 1992 by Congress that can accept funding and create programs that help donors and CDC scientists achieve common goals. The foundation finds funding partners, negotiates funding arrangements, hires staff, manages program budgets, identifies experts, and generates reports to donors.

On its website, the foundation currently lists 37 corporations and 23 foundations that were supporting programs initiated as of July 2000 or that are currently active, including 22 Global Health programs; 8 Promoting Healthy Lifestyles programs; and Research and Education Programs. In 2002-2003, the foundation had revenues of $17.1 million (of which $8.1 million was expended through cost-reimbursement agreements for programs) and expenses of $10.2 million.

Osteoarthritis Initiative Public-Private Consortium

The Osteoarthritis Initiative is a joint venture of NIH and pharmaceutical companies to pool funds and expertise for a public repository of osteoarthritis patient data, radiological information, and biological specimens. Scientists will be able to use this public resource to test much-needed biochemical and imaging markers of disease onset and progression, to further the development of osteoarthritis drugs, and to improve public health. Neither the federal nor private sector alone would be able to develop such a resource.

---

[14]NIH Policy Manual, Chapter 1135, "Gifts Administration," Part E5, "Receipt and Acceptance of Gifts." See www.od.nih.gov/oma/manualchapters/management/1135/main.html.

Scientists, health care providers, and drug companies need biochemical and imaging markers of the progression of osteoarthritis in order to diagnose, monitor, and develop and implement treatments for this condition more accurately than current methods of evaluating disease progression—such as x-rays and pain and function assessments—can. The data and specimen repository will establish standards of disease onset and progression against which potential biochemical and imaging markers can be evaluated. This ultimately will facilitate clinical trials of promising agents.

Four clinical centers and a data coordinating center were chosen after competitive peer review in July 2002 of applications submitted in response to two Requests for Proposals Applications (RFPs). The clinical centers are at the University of Maryland School of Medicine, the Ohio State University, the University of Pittsburgh, and the Memorial Hospital of Rhode Island. The data coordinating center is at the University of California, San Francisco. The recruitment of 5,000 participants, who will be followed for five years, began in February 2004.

The initiative is coordinated by the National Institute of Arthritis and Musculoskeletal and Skin Diseases (NIAMS) and NIA, with additional support from six other NIH institutes, centers, and offices. The private sector partners are Merck, Novartis Pharmaceuticals Corporation, and Pfizer. The private sector members of the consortium pool their resources through the FNIH along with NIH's funds from the participating institutes and centers. FNIH is providing the management structure and also is recruiting, coordinating, and managing the private sector partners in the consortium. The initiative totals $8 million per year. Approximately 30 percent of the funding is contributed by the private sector partners.

All partners have agreed that clinical data and x-ray information will be freely accessible to qualified scientists everywhere. For other resources that are limited (such as biological specimens), priority will be given to researchers who are studying promising biomarkers that will be made widely available for research and commercial use.

Complementary Federal and Private Funding

In some cases, nonfederal funders do not contribute directly to the federal funding of a research program. Instead, they agree to fund directly certain parts of the program, while the federal agency funds other parts.

Type 1 Diabetes TrialNet

In September 2001 the National Institute of Diabetes & Digestive & Kidney Diseases (NIDDK) established the Type 1 Diabetes TrialNet, with co-sponsorship by the National Institute of Child Health and Human Development (NICHD), NIAID, the Juvenile Diabetes Research Foundation International (JDRF), and the American Diabetes Association ADA). TrialNet is a collaborative network of clinical centers, experts in diabetes and immunology, and specialized laboratories and other facilities.

The purpose of the network is to test new approaches to understanding, preventing, and treating type 1 diabetes. TrialNet will enable rapid preliminary testing of emerging therapeutic strategies for immunoprevention of type 1 diabetes, and the agents that prove most promising can then be quickly moved into larger scale trials. In addition, biological samples and other data collected from trial participants are being placed in repositories for use by many investigators. TrialNet also is formulating surrogate endpoints for diabetes and its complications.

The Type 1 Diabetes TrialNet includes 18 clinical centers. NIH funds the 14 centers in the United States and Canada, while JDRF and ADA fund 4 centers in Europe and Australia.

Supplementation of Federal Funding

Some VHAs supplement, or augment, the funding of federal grantees. Typically, the private funding is used for purposes that the federal funds do not or cannot support. For example, the Charlotte Geyer Foundation provides one-year awards to researchers whose proposals have been reviewed by NCI and were ranked within ten percentage points of the NCI pay line. In theory, this type of supplementation could work both ways—that is, nonfederal funders could send meritorious project proposals to CDMRP for funding once their pay line has been reached. However, because CDMRP's peer review system is one of its unique attributes, it is unlikely that it would be willing to sacrifice its own evaluation of proposals and replace it with that of another group. In either case, overall costs could be decreased if one review process were used by multiple funding sources.

Muscular Dystrophy Research Centers

In October 2003, NIAMS, the National Institute of Neurological Disorders and Stroke, and NICHD collaborated with the Muscular Dystrophy Association (MDA) to fund three new extramural centers for research on the muscular dystrophies. The institutes are funding the three centers—selected through competitive peer review—at $5 million each over five years, and MDA is providing up to $500,000 in supplemental funding per center per year for three years. The centers are located at the University of Pittsburgh, the University of Washington, and the University of Rochester.

Mentored Clinical Scientist Awards in Nephrology

The National Kidney Foundation provides monetary supplements to up to four recipients of Mentored Clinical Scientist Development (K08) Awards from NIDDK, making the awards more attractive by increasing pay.

Piggybacking Arrangements

A number of foundations and charitable organizations fund research proposals that receive peer review ratings that are high, but not high enough to receive federal funding. Through this arrangement, the private funder does not have to review the proposals at the funding cutoff level, 20 to 25 percent of which are successful and bring excellent results.

Pathogenesis and Treatment of Cystic Fibrosis

In 1995, NIDDK, the National Heart, Lung, and Blood Institute (NHLBI), and the Cystic Fibrosis Foundation (CFF) co-sponsored an RFA for R01 grants to conduct basic research on the pathogenesis of cystic fibrosis (CF) and its complications, applied cell and molecular biology research to understand CF better, translational research into new treatments for CF, and clinical research on CF and its potential therapies.

According to the RFA:

> Projects with substantial scientific merit that are not funded by the NIDDK or the NHLBI are eligible for support by the CFF. Principal investigators will be responsible for forwarding copies of their summary statements and applications to the CFF for consideration for this award mechanism.

It is anticipated that approximately 15 awards will be made [by NIH]. An additional $2 million will be committed by CFF to fund applications that are not funded by NIDDK or NHLBI.[15]

Private Nonmonetary Contributions

The Alzheimer's Association is partnering with NIA in a major expansion of the Alzheimer's Disease (AD) Genetics Study, which will focus on volunteers from approximately 1,000 families in which multiple members have experienced late-onset AD. At least three members of each family will be asked to donate blood (for determination of their DNA) and provide medical, demographic, and family history information, in an effort to discover the risk factor genes for late-onset AD. The role of the Alzheimer's Association and its network of local chapters is to inform families about the study and encourage their participation (NIH, 2003). Similarly, CFF played an integral role in Food and Drug Administration (FDA) approval of Pulmozyme in 1993 and of TOBI (tobramycin solution for inhalation) in 1997 by assisting in the recruitment of clinical trial participants.[16]

---

[15] RFA-DK-95-006.

[16] See www.cff.org/publications/files/cfinsidespreads.pdf.

CONCLUSION

Federal agencies that support R&D use a variety of mechanisms to leverage other funding. Most of these mechanisms fall into two categories. One set of mechanisms relies on requirements that awardees pay a portion of the costs of the project from nonfederal sources. This is called cost sharing or matching. The other set of mechanisms consists of voluntary collaborations that are made between federal agencies and nonfederal donors in supporting specific research initiatives of mutual interest.

Cost-sharing or matching requirements are commonly used by agencies when industry involvement is desired for a project and industry stands to gain from the effort. These are typically technology development-oriented projects, often involving university-industry research centers.

Cost sharing is usually not required in programs that support basic research and that are conducted by individual investigators or small research teams. NIH does not require matching except for several small challenge grant programs and facility construction projects. NSF requires a nominal 1 percent cost sharing on investigator-initiated awards, although it expects cost sharing of between 10 percent and 30 percent in its center programs and up to 50 percent for instrumentation and facilities awards.

Voluntary co-funding and other forms of partnering have become more common. Some agencies—NIH and CDC—have mechanisms for accepting private funds that augment appropriated funds. These ventures are formed one by one as federal agencies and nonfederal funders see opportunities to leverage their funds by collaborating. These collaborations are unpredictable and take time to organize, and because each partnership is unique, a great deal of effort is required on the part of federal program officers. As such, there must be clear perceived potential benefit for each party to commit the requisite time and resources.

REFERENCES

COGR (Council on Governmental Relations). 2003. Report of the Working Group on the Cost of Doing Business. [On-line.] Available: www.cogr.edu/docs/codb final 6-02-03.doc [accessed June 30, 2004].

DOE (Department of Energy). 2004. Financial Assistance Announcement of Funding Opportunity, Clean Coal Power Initiative, DE-PS26-04NT42061. [On-line.] Available: www.fossil.energy.gov/programs/powersystems/cleancoal/ccpi/ccpi_sol_round2.pdf [accessed July 28, 2004].

Feller I. 1997. *Matching Fund and Cost-Sharing Experiences of U.S. Research Universities: Final Report to the National Science Foundation*. Bethesda, MD: COSMOS Corporation.

Goldman CA, Williams T. 2000. *Paying for University Research Facilities and Administration*. MR-1135-1-OSTP. Santa Monica, CA: RAND. [On-line.] Available: www.rand.org/publications/MR/MR1135.1/ [accessed June 30, 2004].

NASA (National Aeronautics and Space Administration). n.d. *Guidance for the Preparation and Submission of Unsolicited Proposals*. [On-line.] Available: ec.msfc.nasa.gov/hq/library/unsold-Prop.html [accessed May 13, 2004].

NIH (National Institutes of Health). 2003. "National Institute on Aging Steps Up Major New Initiative on Alzheimer's Disease Genetics" (press release). [On-line.] Available: www.nia.nih.gov/news/pr/2003/1021a.htm [accessed August 2, 2004].

NSF (National Science Foundation). 1999. Important Notice 124, Implementation of the New NSF Cost Sharing Policy. [On-line.] Available: www.nsf.gov/pubs/1999/iin124/iin124.htm [accessed May 13, 2004].

NSF. 2002a. *Grant Policy Manual*, Chapter III, Section 330, Cost Sharing and Matching. [On-line.] Available: www.nsf.gov/pubs/2002/nsf02151/gpm3/htm [accessed May 7, 2004].

NSF. 2002b. *National Science Foundation Policy Statement on Cost Sharing*. NSB 02-188. [On-line.] Available: www.nsf.gov/bfa/dga/policy/docs/cspolicy_1102.pdf [accessed May 7, 2004].

NSF. 2004. "U.S. Academic R&D Continues to Grow as More Universities and Colleges Expand Their R&D Activities" (NSF InfoBrief). NSF 04-319. Arlington, VA: National Science Foundation, Division of Science Resources Statistics. [On-line.] Available: www.nsf.gov/sbe/srs/infbrief/nsf04319/start.htm [accessed June 30, 2004].

U.S Army Research Office. 2003. Broad Agency Announcement DAAD19-03-R-0005, Institute for Collaborative Biotechnologies. February. [On-line.] Available: www.aro.army.mil/biotech/ [accessed May 17, 2004].

4

Assessment of Alternative Sources and Mechanisms of Nonfederal Support

Chapter 3 presented a two-by-two typology of alternative funding mechanisms and provided examples of nonfederal support for federal research projects for each typology category, with additional examples presented in Appendix A. Most of the examples were clustered in two of the typology cells: (1) mandatory cost sharing or matching by recipients of awards and (2) voluntary collaborations, or partnerships, between federal agencies and other funders, nonfederal and federal. Currently the Congressionally Directed Medical Research Program (CDMRP) requires grantees to share costs by providing the facilities and equipment to conduct the proposed research or training project, representing a small percentage of the costs, and the committee discussed the possible effects on CDMRP and grantees of raising the amount of mandated cost sharing and matching. The committee then discussed the impact of the second approach—the development of collaborations, or partnerships, with nonfederal funders such as companies, foundations, and states—on CDMRP and those who might participate in these partnerships with the program.

POTENTIAL ADVANTAGES AND DISADVANTAGES OF COST SHARING AND MATCHING REQUIREMENTS

Mandatory cost-sharing or matching requirements have a number of potential advantages and disadvantages for funders and grantees. The primary potential advantage for both parties is that cost-sharing provisions may stretch or conserve limited program funds, allowing more projects to be supported and more support to be dedicated to particular efforts. Scarcity of funds is, in fact, often thought to be a motivation for imposing this requirement even though some federal agencies have issued policies that prohibit the use of cost sharing or matching only to stretch program budgets. According to a Department of Health and Human Services Grants Policy Directive, "Matching or cost sharing may not be required through administrative action solely as a means of offsetting budget reductions" (DHHS, 1999).

Cost-sharing and matching requirements also can serve to leverage new sources of funding. Indeed, some organizations may specifically orient their giving to take advantage of such arrangements. According to a report on trends in U.S. funding for biomedical research, for example, the Pew Charitable Trusts "have attempted to identify a place within the biomedical research funding community where their support can be effectively leveraged to achieve the greatest impact" (University of California, 1996). Other programs, such as the California Breast Cancer Research Program (see Appendix A), have adopted the same strategy.

Cost sharing or matching also can help assure real commitment to projects by participants, which may be particularly true for technology development programs, where cost sharing can provide some assurance that a company views a project as a promising one. The Advanced Technology Program of the National Institute of Standards and Technology, for example, imposes strict cost-sharing requirements for its grantees (see Appendix A). A National Research Council assessment (2001) notes that this feature keeps the program anchored in the market economy and focused on efficiency and the bottom line. It also provides a mechanism for weeding out unpromising research approaches.

However, a number of potential negative effects of the cost-sharing or matching mechanism also have been identified (Feller, 1997, 2000a, 2000b; Hardy, 2000; Seligman, 2000). It might, for example, shift funding from other related projects and thus not yield a net benefit to the advancement of knowledge. In addition, the pot of money available for research on a given topic would be unlikely to change if CDMRP imposed cost-sharing or matching requirements; what might change, however, is the decisionmaking process of the organizations responsible for administering research funding. If organizations—for example, those dedicated to supporting research on a specific disease—perceive that investigations will no longer be supported by CDMRP unless they provide funds, they may divert resources from other projects to meet this requirement.

Cost sharing or matching also would impose additional costs on applicants, their institutions, and CDMRP, because applicant and institutional costs include those incurred in the process of identifying and accounting for sources of matching funds. This entails having more staff and spending more time preparing funding proposals. Often, the principal investigator loses valuable research time in order to participate in proposal preparation. For CDMRP, this would mean an increase in proposal review time and effort as well as the need to provide auditing to ensure that the cost sharing is legitimate and not doubly counted as cost sharing for other federal grants. However, it is difficult to estimate the precise scale and impact of these costs, because hard data in this area are lacking.

Mandating cost sharing or matching also would inject financial criteria into the peer review process, the most direct consequence of which would be that some high-quality proposals may not receiving funding or may never be submitted because of a lack of adequate matching funds, while some lower quality proposals for which matching funds are available might succeed. A study of cost sharing at the National Science Foundation (NSF) by Feller (2000a) showed that open-ended cost sharing resulted in bidding wars, and recent NSF Inspector General reports have found that as a result, grantees often were unable to deliver the cost sharing they had optimistically bid to win the award.

If cost sharing or matching were mandated, universities with significant institutional resources would have a competitive advantage, as they may have an office specifically intended to identify potential sources of funding and to administer policies to obtain such funding. Cohen et al. (1998) note that several universities now maintain such offices to administer technology transfer and licensing in order to facilitate funding relationships. In addition, Larson and Brahmakulam (2002) found that "partnership friendly" policies make a difference in the ability of universities to attract cooperative funding. The development of policies that promote cost sharing or matching also takes a commitment on the part of the institution that may be more difficult to make when resources are scarce.

Seligman (2000) suggests that cost-sharing requirements present an opportunity for some institutions to improve their standing in the ranks of research recipients by buying their way into grants that they might otherwise be unlikely to receive. Furthermore, economies of scale may provide an advantage to larger and more financially secure institutions, including larger indirect cost recovery funds from which to draw.

Mandated cost sharing or matching would give universities in states with aggressive economic development or other research promotion programs a competitive advantage. Some states are explicit in their intent to use funds in this matter. For example, the Arkansas Research Matching Fund states that its purpose is "[t]o raise the national ranking of Arkansas' research performance and to be competitive in our economic and educational endeavors by investing in research and research infrastructure" (Arkansas Science and Technology Authority, 2000).

These arrangements could distort the priorities of awardee institutions by imposing financial obligations that detract from other university missions, such as instructional programs. This concern is expressed by a number of sources, including a draft DOD cost-sharing policy; however, the committee did not identify any studies that substantiate it. Bienenstock (2000) was told anecdotally by the president of a southern public university that, because of the importance of research in maintaining faculty vitality, he felt pressured to divert funding from the humanities to provide cost sharing to secure research grants.

CDMRP priorities, which are set by each program's Integration Panel, might be distorted if it is easier to fund some types of activities than others. A primary concern in this regard, as discussed elsewhere in the report, is that applied research is far more likely than basic research to attract the interest of industries that can supply funding—a direct consequence of the for-profit sector making the rational choice to seek to benefit from its investment by obtaining preferential access to new knowledge. There is some literature relevant to this issue that addresses the more general question of whether economic pressures have resulted in a shift from basic to applied work in academic research. Cohen et al. (1998) note that universities are pushing toward greater funding from industry and observe that this drive may well be a reflection of the decreasing support for research offered by government sources. Although the researchers argue that industry sponsorship goes preferentially to applied research, there are no data that show that this shifts academic work toward applied research. In fact, the National Science Board (NSB) in its examination of trends in researchers' activities from 1993 to 1999 (2002), found that the decrease in the basic research component of those activities was modest (although statistically significant), from 61.9 percent to 59.9 percent.

AGENCY EXPERIENCES WITH COST SHARING

The experiences of NSF with cost sharing are instructive. In the early 1990s, NSF (and other federal agencies) began to ratchet up cost-sharing requirements, and the aggregate impact on universities began to cause many of the problems outlined above. After a survey by Irwin Feller in 1997 on the *Matching Fund and Cost-Sharing Experiences of U.S. Research Universities* documented these problems, NSF adopted a new, more restrictive policy on cost sharing in 1999 (Feller, 1997). The new NSF policy specified that:

- Cost sharing is an eligibility criterion, not a review criterion (that is, voluntary cost sharing beyond the required amount stated in the solicitation is not supposed to be a factor in review).
- Only statutory cost sharing (1 percent) is required for unsolicited proposals (which includes those responsive to general program announcements).
- Cost sharing that exceeds 1 percent must be clearly stated in the solicitation.
- If the proposed cost of the project is reduced, the level of cost sharing must be reduced accordingly (thus preventing the shifting of costs to the recipient).

The policy statement on cost sharing also provided criteria for imposing higher cost sharing:

> In addition to the statutory requirements [of 1 percent], NSF can require cost sharing when we believe there is tangible benefit to the award recipient(s) (normally beyond the immediate term or scope of the NSF-supported activity). Benefit is defined in terms of capacity building, potential dollar revenues, time frames, or third party users. NSF-funded activities which are characterized by

> such benefits are awards for infrastructure-building purposes (instrumentation/equipment/centers/facilities) or for awards where there is clear potential to make profit or generate income (e.g., curriculum development) (NSB, 1999).

Another impetus for the new NSF policy was a series of reports from the Office of Inspector General (OIG) of NSF about the problems it was finding in university accounting for cost sharing. The NSF OIG was concerned because in FY 2000, for example, NSF awards required cost sharing totaling more than a half billion dollars. "Given the large amount of these commitments, the failure to honor cost-sharing obligations or to keep proper accounts can have serious consequences for NSF's awards" (NSF, 2003a).

The NSF OIG identified the keeping of cost-sharing commitments as one of the 10 most serious management and performance challenges facing NSF beginning in FY 2001, following findings of "overvalued and unsupported cost sharing" at 2 campuses of a western state university system in 2000 and 2001. The OIG concluded that cost sharing was overstated to make proposals more competitive, but that the institutions subsequently were unable to show how much was actually provided (NSF-OIG, 2002).The OIG then conducted two audits to gauge the extent of cost-sharing problems and whether they were systemic. One audit covered five additional campuses at the same western state university system, while the second was of eight educational institutions that had pledged $500,000 or more of cost sharing. In most cases, the universities could not substantiate some of the cost sharing. In 2003, the NSF Inspector General wrote NSF and NSB that "our past audit work indicates that many awardees do not adequately account for or substantiate the value of cost-share expenditures, raising questions about whether required contributions are actually being made" (NSF, 2003b).

On December 28, 2000, in response to a 1999 report of the National Science and Technology Council, *Renewing the Government-University Partnership*, the President issued Executive Order 13185, "To Strengthen the Federal Government-University Research Partnership." The Executive Order presented a list of principles, one of which was that "Agency cost-sharing policies and practices must be transparent." DOD responded by drafting a policy, *Cost Sharing in DOD Research Programs Using Assistance Instruments*, as part of the DOD series of administrative instruction.[1] The instruction, which has not been formally issued, said that while DOD does not have a general requirement of cost sharing in its research grant programs, program offices could use cost sharing in individual programs on a case-by-case basis if they follow procedures to ensure that its use is appropriate.[2] Inappropriate use of cost-sharing requirements could be unfair to

---

[1]See www.acq.osd.mil/ddre/research/draftcostsharing.pdf.

[2]DOD policies for R&D contracts prohibit cost sharing unless there is a reasonable probability of potential commercial applications (subparagraph E1.6 of DOD Instruction 5000.1, The Defense Acquisition System, May 12, 2003).

those conducting research, for example, if it stimulated competitive cost-share bidding, and it could create financial hardship and draw funds for research that otherwise would go to undergraduate education or the broader research infrastructure (also interests of DOD). It also could disqualify some proposals that may be technically outstanding, but that are submitted by applicants who are unable to participate in cost sharing.

The DOD instruction specified that cost sharing should be used only when there is a policy basis for it: "Budget augmentation is never to be used as a reason to require cost sharing." A policy basis is either a statutory requirement for cost sharing or the existence of projects that would generate benefits for the entity that performed the research beyond DOD-related benefits. Cost sharing is especially appropriate in dual-use research, for example, "not only because the performers should benefit financially from commercialization, but also because cost sharing is strong evidence of their judgment that the technology is likely to be commercially viable."

Although DOD has not issued the draft guidance for cost sharing in assistance agreements, the Undersecretary of Defense for Acquisition and Technology has strongly discouraged cost sharing in R&D contracts: "Contractors should not be encouraged or required to supplement DOD appropriations by bearing a portion of defense contract costs. . ." (Aldridge, 2001).[3]

Other agencies also limit cost sharing on research projects to instances when the recipient will gain some monetary benefit from the project—that is, for technology development projects. For example, the National Aeronautics and Space Administration (NASA) *Guidance for the Preparation and Submission of Unsolicited Proposals* says:

> By statute, cost sharing is usually required on contracts for basic or applied research projects resulting from unsolicited proposals However, colleges and universities need not propose cost sharing since their activities generally do not produce benefits that can be measured as having significance apart from the benefit intrinsic in conducting research for NASA.[4]

NASA grants and cooperative agreements do not require cost sharing by institutions of higher education, hospitals, or other nonprofit organizations, and it is only required of commercial firms if they are "expected to receive substantial compensating benefits for performance of the work."[5]

---

[3]"The only exception to this policy would be unusual situations where there is a reasonable probability of a potential commercial application related to the research and development effort."

[4]National Aeronautics and Space Administration. *Guidance for the Preparation and Submission of Unsolicited Proposals*. See ec.msfc.nasa.gov/hq/library/unsold-Prop.html.

[5]National Aeronautics and Space Administration. Section A, Part 1260—Grants and Cooperative Agreements, in *NASA Grant Policy Book*. See ec.msfc.nasa.gov/hq/granta.doc.

The Department of Energy (DOE) has a similar policy of not imposing cost sharing on basic research.

> The decision as to whether an acquisition or assistance agreement will include either a cost-sharing or cost-participation provision, respectively, is made on a case-by-case basis. Normally, DOE will fully fund the early phases of basic research and development programs. However, subsequent phases of those programs, which provide the performer with present or future economic benefits through commercialization, will require some form of cost-sharing or cost-participation.[6]

In conclusion, although matching fund requirements at first glance appear to be a good way to leverage funds, for several reasons they may not in fact expand the amount of research conducted in a particular area. First, matching funds may be diverted from other research projects, and some highly promising research may go unfunded because of a lack of matching funds, or the match itself may reduce the total number of projects and therefore the number of ideas that are funded. Second, the matching requirements are not free from demands on time and resources on the part of principal investigators and institutional research administrators, who must line up donors, plan the project, and prepare a more complex application. Involving multiple funders also may further dilute the focus of the research because they may have different objectives. In addition, opportunity costs may become involved, because the time researchers must allocate to fundraising is time not spent conducting research. This may have the effect of hindering important scientific advances. It also may be the case that imposing matching requirements could result in better known investigators attracting more funding than investigators who may be less prominent. Along the same lines, wealthier institutions that have greater means to provide matching funds may attract more support than other entities that have fewer resources. Finally, as mentioned earlier, both the recipient institution and CDMRP would have to expand their staffs to audit the matching funds in order to ensure that they are legitimate and not counted as matching on another federal grant.

VOLUNTARY COLLABORATIONS

The April 2004 two-day workshop convened by this committee and the review of research on public-private collaborations in R&D prepared for the committee by Andrew Toole and Anwar Naseem (see Appendix D) focused on the incentives for nonfederal funders to pool or coordinate their resources with

---

[6]Department of Energy. *Guide for the Submission of Unsolicited Proposals.* See professionals.pr.doe.gov/ma5/MA-5Web.nsf/WebAttachments/UnsolicitedProposal/$File/UnsolicitedProposal.pdf.

CDMRP. For-profit firms, universities, foundations and other charities, and state governments have different goals and constituencies, and they operate under different norms of behavior, laws and regulations, and other constraints. Thus, it could be asked why they would wish to collaborate. "The answer, according to the literature, is that each party gets something they value out of the arrangement" (Toole and Naseem, Appendix D, p. 143). That is, the advantages of such an arrangement are that each participant can leverage the other and can expect to see a benefit from the collaboration, which can achieve a critical mass by pooling resources for a large-scale project or by creating a synergy that results in the whole becoming greater than the sum of its parts.

Cooperative R&D consortia are prevalent in other sectors, especially the microelectronics sector, to support generic pre-competitive research, going back to the Electric Power Research Institute in 1972, the Gas Research Institute in 1976, the Microelectronics Center of North Carolina in 1980, and the Semiconductor Research Corporation and the Microelectronics and Computer Technology Corporation in 1982. The National Cooperative Research Act was passed in 1984 to exempt such consortia from antitrust laws. These and later consortia, such as SEMATECH, support the development of technologies that can be used by all members, and they often develop technology "roadmaps" to guide research funding.

In a different approach, the Central Intelligence Agency (CIA) has established its own venture capital enterprise, InQTel. InQTel's mission is to stimulate the development of leading-edge technologies that might be useful to the CIA by investing in promising companies.

Public-private R&D consortia are less common in the biopharmaceutical sector, although there are some examples, such as the Osteoarthritis Initiative, which is described in Chapter 3. The Mouse Sequencing Consortium and the Alzheimer's Disease Neuroimaging Initiative include for-profit companies and foundations that are co-funding the functional equivalent of generic pre-competitive research—the mouse genome sequence and biomarkers that can be used to evaluate disease progression in clinical trials.

Public-private partnerships (PPPs) have been growing rapidly in the international sector, facilitated by several large foundations with an interest in international health, such as the Wellcome Trust and the Bill and Melinda Gates Foundation. One of these, the Global Alliance for TB Drug Development, was the subject of a presentation by its CEO at the April 2004 workshop. Most of the international PPPs for R&D focus on product development, such as vaccines, drugs, diagnostics, and microbicides (Widdus, 2003).[7] Their strategy is to fund key steps in the process between research and delivery that the private sector alone is not funding because of the risks of high costs and small markets. These

[7]Other international public-private partnerships focus on product access through distribution of low cost therapeutics (Widdus, 2003).

steps include target identification and characterization, identification of hit compounds, converting hit compounds to leads, pre-clinical research, Phase I, II, and III clinical trials, and regulatory approval. Funding of product development PPPs totals nearly $1 billion, of which more than $700 million has been committed by the Gates Foundation (Kettler, 2003).

These ventures are focused on the development of products, platform technologies, research tools, and research resources such as databases rather than basic research. PPPs for funding research are less common, although there are examples. Some foundations and public charities—for example, the Cystic Fibrosis Foundation, the Muscular Dystrophy Association, and the Juvenile Diabetes Research Foundation International—have co-funded or supplemented National Institutes of Health (NIH) research and research training grants, but the amounts of funding are relatively small. An exception is the Avon Foundation, which recently pledged $20 million to the National Cancer Institute (NCI) for a program of clinical research grants (see Box 4-1).

On the other hand, there are a number of possible disadvantages to these collaborations:

- Collaborations to stretch program resources might distort CDMRP's priorities because only certain kinds of activities are likely to be of interest to the other funding sources with the deepest pockets, such as industry and state economic development programs. These will tend to be research and related efforts (i.e., infrastructure and training) that have near-term commercial possibilities and not those that the majority of CDMRP's budget currently supports—i.e., exploratory and other early-stage research projects).
- Program administration may be more complicated because collaborators usually will want to have a say in program direction.
- To the extent the activities will result in generic or precompetitive knowledge that can be exploited by others ("free riders"), or produce trainees that might go to work for competitors, attracting industry funds will be more difficult. Collaborating companies will want off-setting compensation, such as faster or more extensive access to research results, or a larger share in the intellectual property rights resulting from the research.
- Universities in geographic regions that are already institutionally rich with R&D organizations and related functions will have a competitive advantage in forming research funding collaborations. This would include universities in California's Silicon Valley, on Massachusetts' Route 128, in North Carolina's Research Triangle Park, near NIH in Maryland, near pharmaceutical firms in the Delaware Valley, around Austin, Texas, or near San Diego, California (DeVol et al., 2004).

According to Toole and Naseem (Appendix D), government sees R&D collaborations as a mechanism to leverage limited financial resources and, in some

BOX 4-1
Avon Foundation-NCI "Progress for Patients" Awards Program

The corporate foundation of Avon Products, Inc., established the Avon Breast Cancer Crusade in the United States in 1993 to raise funds for breast cancer medical research, education, and support services. Most of the funds come from annual three-day fundraising walks, the Avon Breast Cancer 3-Day, and the proceeds of special Avon Crusade Pink Ribbon products sold by Avon sales representatives.

The Avon Foundation awards competitively peer reviewed grants in research areas that have high potential but that are underfunded by other sources. Examples include research on new screening technologies; prevention and risk reduction strategies; therapeutic vaccines; and the role of environmental factors and genetic susceptibility in the causation of breast cancer (Avon Foundation, 2004).

In the past, the Avon Foundation solicited proposals from and made grants to academic health centers and other nonprofits on the basis of a peer review process it arranged. In 2002, Avon pledged $20 million to NCI to fund breast cancer research over five years through a competition open to institutions with NCI cancer center and/or SPORE (Specialized Programs of Research Excellence) grants. Called the Avon Foundation-NCI "Progress for Patients" Awards for Early Phase Clinical Interventions in Breast Cancer, the program is intended to provide a rapid means to support novel and promising Phase I and II clinical trials and studies focusing on risk assessment or validation of biomarkers in human subjects (NCI-Avon, 2003).

In this partnership, NCI conducts the application and review process and administers the awards and most of the indirect costs for the awards. Avon is responsible for supplying funds to NCI for the direct costs and up to 10 percent of the indirect costs of the awards and can take advantage of NCI's peer review process and award administration system to save those costs. For NCI, as an official explained at the announcement of the first awards in October 2002:

> It's a cost savings because instead of paying $2.5 million for grants through our SPOREs, We're only paying $600,000 and saving about $2 million every six months...We are in a situation where everyone is winning because we are providing our expertise and a private foundation like Avon is providing their funding and insight. Otherwise, we would not have been able to make all these awards possible (NCI, 2002).

According to the president of Avon Products:

> As a company for women, Avon is committed to corporate social responsibility and to the breast cancer cause, one of the most important issues in women's health.... With this latest gift [of $20 million], we are especially proud to initiate a unique public-private partnership with the National Cancer Institute. (Avon Products, 2001)

In the first round, Avon provided $1.99 million and NCI $660,000 for six two-year awards. To date, the program has made 19 awards, and NCI is reviewing 32 proposals for another round of funding in the summer of 2004.

cases, unique research capabilities to achieve social goals such as (1) increasing industrial competitiveness; (2) fostering economic growth by overcoming market failures in R&D markets; and (3) meeting agency-specific mission-oriented goals through cost- and risk-sharing. One of the risks facing government agencies involved in public-private R&D collaborations is the problem of measuring results, because the effects of research are often indirect and may occur years in the future. Another major concern is the status of public opinion and trust relationships between public agencies and citizens, because private partners may appear to be dominant and to be using public resources for their own gain.

For-profit firms engage in R&D collaborations because such research partnerships have potential benefits. They are a cost-effective alternative to paying for in-house research capacity, and they improve the effectiveness of a firm's strategic management by enabling it to see how a technology is developing without having to pay the full costs of such an effort. Collaborations in generic or precompetitive research, when they involve other firms, mitigate the problem of underinvestment in R&D, which can happen when firms, acting alone, do not wish to pay for research that could be exploited by competitors. Firms also want access to leading university scientists, federal laboratory scientists, and students trained in the latest methods and tools who can be recruited subsequently for employment.

The risks of collaborations for for-profit firms include those of losing proprietary information and gaining incomplete intellectual property rights when new technologies are developed jointly. Firms also have to worry about recouping their investments, given that industrial research generally proceeds over a much shorter period than does academic research.

IMPACTS OF ALTERNATIVES ON THE CURRENT PROGRAM

Although the scientific community was initially skeptical about CDMRP's location in DOD and the participation of consumers in its peer review and priority-setting processes, it has been demonstrated to be a program that has been efficiently managed and scientifically productive, and it has become a valuable component of the nation's health research enterprise (IOM, 1997). At the committee's April 2004 workshop, consumer representatives cautioned that great care should be taken to ensure that changes in the program intended to leverage funding do not damage the features that have made it efficient and cost effective, driven by scientific priorities, and scientifically productive (Atkins, 2004; Kolker, 2004; Visco, 2004). Some of these features are low administrative costs, an effective two-tier peer review system, and program priorities that are focused on new investigators and basic research, including exploratory grants.

Administrative Costs

Currently, compared with most other government programs, CDMRP has a relatively low administrative overhead of approximately 6 percent. Although increased cost-sharing requirements would impose costs chiefly on applicants and awardees—in terms of time or diversion of recipient resources—it also would require more DOD staff in order to ensure that cost-sharing requirements are met and to arrange and maintain relationships with the other funders. Establishing a foundation to plan collaborative programs and solicit funding from nonfederal sources would only add to overhead costs.

Peer Review

CDMRP has used the two-tier review system recommended in the 1993 IOM report to ensure that scientific quality and program relevance are the main determinants of the distribution of funds. Increased cost sharing would need to be carefully designed to ensure that the peer review system is not distorted, for example, by discouraging proposals from institutions that do not have access to many cost-sharing resources or by creating a bidding war.

If CDMRP adopts the strategy of accepting donations from pharmaceutical or biotechnology companies to expand the pool of grants for a particular program of mutual interest, the funding should be distributed through the regular peer review process to recipients that present the best proposals in terms of technical excellence and program relevance. The funding should not be earmarked for specific projects.

Program Priorities

Currently, the majority of funding appropriated to CDMRP supports new investigators and exploratory basic, translational, and clinical research—activities that industry is less likely to want to co-fund than those that may be closer to commercial development. Although foundations and charities do fund basic and exploratory research, and should be encouraged to collaborate, they have relatively few resources compared with industry or the federal government. The easiest way to maximize nonfederal funding would be to change program priorities to emphasize the development and testing of diagnostics, therapeutics, medical devices, and other efforts to develop commercial products. However, the advisability of such a shift should be carefully considered, given the amount of funding that industry and other federal agencies already devote to such activities, especially considering the great need for additional basic, especially exploratory, research in understanding the diseases addressed by CDMRP.

Potential Consequences of Collaboration with For-Profit Firms

The consequences of a government agency collaboration with for-profit firms could include the imposition of secrecy on the scientific process, possible delays and bias in the reporting of research results, the shifting of research priorities toward near-term development, and financial conflicts of interest for both the research institutions and the individual researchers (Campbell et al., 2004). Studies of academic institutions collaborating with industry—which provide a close analogy to government-industrial partnerships—have shown that academic institutions can face numerous challenges: conflicts of interest can emerge for faculty interested in benefiting financially from their university research; increased secrecy and other restrictions can limit dissemination of industrial research results; time spent on commercial research can reduce faculty commitments to the university; and use of students on privately funded research can divert resources and place limits on the ability of students to communicate the results of their work (see studies cited by Campbell et al., 2004).

NIH has recognized the issues that might arise in public-private ventures. In 1994, NIH issued guidelines on *Developing Sponsored Research Agreements: Considerations for Recipients of NIH Research Grants and Contracts*, which were intended

> to provide Recipients with issues and points to consider in developing sponsored research agreements with commercial entities, where such agreements may include research activities which are fully or partially funded by NIH. The intent is to assist recipients in ensuring that these agreements comply with the requirements of the Bayh-Dole Act and NIH funding agreements while upholding basic principles of academic freedom.[8]

These guidelines focus on the preservation of academic freedom, the timely dissemination of research results, and permissible amounts of private support both absolutely and as a percentage of the recipient's total research funding.

In addition, in 1997 the Centers for Disease Control and Prevention (CDC) issued *Guidance for Collaboration with the Private Sector,*[9] and CDC and the CDC Foundation have developed *Joint Guidelines for Co-Sponsorship Arrangements*, a document that contains a list of "red flag issues" that arise if the answers to certain questions are unsatisfactory. These issues must be resolved or arrangements must be made to manage them before a collaborative activity is undertaken. The questions include the following:

---

[8]See ott.od.nih.gov/NewPages/text-com.htm. In 2003, the National Heart, Lung, and Blood Institute issued revised guidelines for "Third Party Involvement in NHLBI-Supported Clinical Trials and Other Population-Based Studies: Awardee/Contractor Third Party Related Issues." See www.nhlbi.nih.gov/funding/policies/thirdparty.htm.

[9]See www.cdc.gov/od/foia/policies/collabor.htm.

- Does the potential co-sponsorship arrangement appear to lack an identifiable, substantial public health benefit?
- Does the potential co-sponsorship arrangement appear to lack a clear, identifiable, substantial leadership role for CDC?
- Is the nonfederal entity a "prohibited source" under the Standards of Ethical Conduct for Employees of the Executive Branch?
- Has the nonfederal entity indicated that its funding is revocable or contingent on any action by CDC other than actions described in the proposal documents (including, for example, the . . . participation of certain individuals in the event, etc.)?
- Has the nonfederal entity requested exclusivity in the co-sponsorship arrangement or otherwise suggested a structure which could create the impression of a "brand affiliation," endorsement, or other form of advertising for the nonfederal entity?
- Does the potential project create any real or perceived conflict of interest (financial or personal) for staff or Board members of CDC, CDC Foundation, or their families?
- Will the anticipated outcomes of the co-sponsorship arrangement likely lead to direct monetary benefit for the nonfederal entity?
- Does the potential project follow the requirements for independence and objectivity of scientific judgment as set forth in CDC's *Guidelines for Collaboration with the Private Sector*?

Universities have also developed guidelines for collaborating with external parties. The University of California, for example, issued guiding principles to govern "research relationship with governmental agencies, nonprofit foundations, and industry." The principles include open dissemination of research results; commitment to students; public benefit; legal integrity; and avoidance of conflicts of interest.[10]

DOD should consider the relevancy and applicability of these guidelines in developing a set that could be applied to CDMRP collaborations.

CHANGES IN FEDERAL LAWS AND REGULATIONS REQUIRED BY ALTERNATIVE FUNDING SOURCES AND MECHANISMS

DOD has the authority to award grants, cooperative agreements, and contracts to for-profit enterprises, states, and consortia as well as to universities and other nonprofit research institutions. It also has the authority to require cost sharing on grants, cooperative agreements, and contracts, at least to the extent that the other party or parties are expected to benefit. But DOD lacks adequate

[10]See www.ucop.edu/california-institutes/pdf/factsheets.pdf.

authority to accept conditional contributions that the donors may want to direct to an extramural grant program such as CDMRP. It also cannot solicit private funds and does not have a means to overcome that restriction, such as establishing a foundation that could accept funding for the agency (as was done for NIH with the Foundation for the National Institutes of Health [FNIH] or for CDC, with the CDC Foundation). Unlike NIH, CDC, or NSF, however, DOD has special authority to make awards that are not subject to conditions that apply to federal grants, cooperative agreements, and contracts, such as Bayh-Dole intellectual property provisions, and this authority could be delegated to CDMRP to make it easier to co-fund projects with for-profit firms that have technologies of interest to CDMRP.[11]

Gift Authority

One mechanism for securing nonfederal funding for CDMRP would be to accept voluntary contributions from foundations, companies, state governments, and other funders of medical research to enlarge a specific CDMRP grant program. NIH, for example, has the authority under Sections 231 and 405 of the Public Health Service Act to accept conditional gifts for study, investigation, or research and other purposes [42 U.S.C. 238(a)]. Currently, under 10 U.S.C. 2601, which authorizes general gift funds, the purpose of contributions to the U.S. Army or DOD cannot be specified by the donor except for hospitals, schools, and other health, education, and welfare activities. Other donations must be unconditional and appropriated by Congress before they can be used.

In order for CDMRP to accept nonfederal funds in support of a project or program, DOD would need statutory authorization to accept contributions from nonfederal donors for a specific purpose—for example, to fund grants for research on a particular disease. Based on the NIH and CDC experience, however, the amounts of nonfederal funding would be very small compared with federal funding.

Dedicated Fundraising Foundation

A nonprofit foundation could be used to solicit funds for CDMRP programs. Such a foundation would be needed because, even if CDMRP were authorized to accept contributions, federal employees may not actively seek them to augment appropriated funds [36 Comp. Gen. 268,269 (1956)]. As mentioned earlier, some agencies, such as NIH (42 U.S.C. 290b) and CDC (42 U.S.C. 280e-11), have foundations with staffs that seek donors for agency programs (see Box 4-2). To establish a similar foundation for CDMRP, Congress would need to create a

---

[11]The Director of NIH recently received "other transactions" authority for expending his Director's Discretionary Fund, which is $45 million in FY 2004.

BOX 4-2
FNIH

FNIH was chartered by Congress in 1990 as a means for NIH to establish relationships with and raise funds from private partners in academia, philanthropy, and industry. FNIH is a 501(c)(3) nonprofit organization that has raised $258 million in private dollars, $200 million of which came from a single grant received from the Bill and Melinda Gates Foundation in 2003 to establish and administer a new program, the Grand Challenges in Global Health Initiative. Thus far, FNIH has received $3.5 million from appropriated funds for operating costs.

Currently, the foundation manages 39 programs, mostly in education, training, and research. In 2000, the foundation was the mechanism for used to pool $30 million from industry and a foundation with NIH funding to establish a Mouse Sequencing Consortium. The consortium was able to sequence the mouse genome in a far shorter time than would have been possible otherwise. Currently, FNIH is managing the private share of the Osteoarthritis Initiative. Three pharmaceutical companies are providing $22 million of the $60 million being spent to create a public database of biomarkers for the progression of osteoarthritis, which will improve research and clinical testing. The foundation also manages the Best Pharmaceuticals for Children Fund, through which corporations, foundations, and interested individuals can partner with the National Institute for Child Health and Human Development to fund clinical studies in pediatric patients. Also currently, FNIH is raising $20 million from pharmaceutical and medical imaging companies as part of a $60 million Alzheimer's Disease neuroimaging program sponsored by the National Institute on Aging, which is providing the other $40 million, the Food and Drug Administration, the Alzheimer's Association, and the Institute for the Study of Aging.

charter for it or expand the authority of the Henry M. Jackson Foundation for the Advancement of Military Medicine.

Grant and Contract Provisions That Concern Some Companies

Grants and cooperative agreements for extramural research are subject to a number of conditions that may deter some commercial firms from doing business with the federal government. Under 10 U.S.C. 2371, the Defense Advanced Research Projects Agency (DARPA) and the military departments (including the U.S. Army) have the authority to enter into transactions other than contracts, grants, and cooperative agreements. Such "other transactions" are exempt from the usual controls and oversight mechanisms set forth in acquisition statutes and the Federal Acquisition Regulation and from laws applying only to contracts, grants, and cooperative agreements. Under this authority, DOD has established

BOX 4-3
Example of a TIA

In 2000, DARPA entered into a TIA with Motorola, Inc., to develop a multichip module sample preparation system for genetic analysis, which could be used for rapid early detection of infection, exposure to biowarfare agents, and general health monitoring. DOD wanted access to Motorola's technology, but Motorola does not accept standard government R&D contracts for research. The TIA permitted Motorola to use its existing accounting systems, which were not compliant with the Federal Acquisition Regulation, and to negotiate other rights important to the company, including alternate dispute resolution procedures, intellectual property rights less stringent than the requirements of the Bayh-Dole Act, and foreign access to technology. In return, Motorola paid $1.5 million of the $4.9 million cost of the project.[a]

[a]"Annual Report on Cooperative Agreements and Other Transactions Entered into during FY2001 under 10 USC 2371." See www.acq.osd.mil/dpap/Docs/FY01RPT.doc.

an assistance instrument called the Technology Investment Agreement (TIA) in which DOD partners with a company or consortium of companies that contribute half or more of the costs. The purpose of TIAs is to increase participation in defense R&D of for-profit firms reluctant to comply with standard grants and contracts regulations, whose requirements or procedures are considered too burdensome, intrusive, or costly. In a TIA, for example, DOD may negotiate less restrictive intellectual property rights than Bayh-Dole requires (see Box 4-3).

TIAs would be most appropriate when CDMRP is trying to stimulate product or technology development with enough commercial promise that a firm or firms would be willing to pay for half the costs. CDMRP can only award and administer TIAs if the Secretary of the Army delegates the authorities in 10 U.S.C. 2371.

SUMMARY

Experience with cost sharing in other federal basic research programs shows that requiring recipients to provide a significant percentage of project costs in order to augment federal funds can impose extra costs on both the recipient and the funder, can have unintended—and often unwanted—consequences (such as discouraging outstanding proposals from researchers at institutions with limited means), and may not substantially increase the total amount of funding in an area of research (or may redirect it from other important uses). Cost sharing is most appropriate when the co-funder receives a tangible benefit, which is much more likely to happen in later-stage research or infrastructure projects than in exploratory research. Yet the greatest strength of CDMRP has been in the earlier stages of research. Thus, while cost sharing can be a valuable and promising approach to pooling resources for a common goal, it is less effective in the context of exploratory research, where outcomes cannot be predicted.

In using cost-sharing mechanisms, CDMRP should ensure that it does not divert funds from other desirable activities, such as other research projects that would have been funded or the instructional programs of universities. In addition, CDMRP should not let expectations of increased nonfederal funding shift the program's scientific priorities away from funding innovative exploratory research, research into disease prevention and causation, and epidemiological studies.

The experience of federal R&D funding agencies with voluntary public-private collaborations generally has been a positive one. Collaborations can leverage research results by achieving synergy, economies of scale, critical mass, or other ways in which the whole becomes greater than the sum of its parts. However, because each collaboration must be individually negotiated, significant costs can be added to the research., as well as additional time, which can delay the start of research. In any case, arranging and maintaining such collaborations require substantial effort, and it is difficult to know, in the long run, how cost effective they will be. However, CDMRP already engages in some collaborations with the private sector and should continue to do so as opportunities arise.

Unlike some other federal research agencies, neither CDMRP nor its parent organization, the U.S. Army Medical Research and Materiel Command, has the authority to receive outside funds to augment its budget for extramural awards. Congress would have to provide for the additional costs of establishing and maintaining a foundation to perform this function. Having this authority would increase opportunities for augmenting funding and entering into collaborative research efforts with the private sector.

REFERENCES

Aldridge EC, Jr. 2001. Contractor Cost Sharing, Memorandum from E.C. Aldridge, Jr., Under Secretary of Defense, to the Secretaries of the Military Departments; Director, Defense Research and Engineering; Directors of Defense Agencies, May 16. [On-line.] Available: www.acq.osd.mil/dpap/Docs/costshare-051601.pdf [accessed July 28, 2004].

Arkansas Science and Technology Authority. 2000. *2000 Annual Report*. [On-line.] Available: asta.ar.gov/fy00ar.html [accessed July 28, 2004].

Atkins R. 2004. Presentation by Dr. Rick Atkins, President and CEO, National Prostate Cancer Coalition, at the workshop held by the Committee on Alternative Funding Strategies for DOD's Peer Reviewed Medical Research Programs. National Academies, Washington, DC, April 26.

Avon Foundation. 2004. 2004 Breast Cancer Funding Guidelines: Improving the Lives of Women and Their Families. [On-line.] Available: www.avoncompany.com/women/ [accessed July 28, 2004].

Avon Products. 2001. Avon Products Foundation Announces Record-Setting Funding for the Fight against Breast Cancer [press release]. [On-line.] Available: www.corporate-ir.net/ireye/ir_site.zhtml?ticker=AVP&script=410&layout=6&item_id=213691 [accessed July 28, 2004].

Bienenstock A. 2000. "Some Thoughts on Cost Sharing." *Research Management Review*, 11(Spring/Summer):9-19.

Campbell EG, Koski G, Blumenthal D. 2004. "The Triple Helix: University, Government, and Industry Relationships in the Life Sciences." Working Paper 04-12. Washington, DC: AEI-Brookings Joint Center for Regulatory Studies.[On-line.] Available: aei-brookings.org/admin/authorpdfs/page.php?id=1000 [accessed June 30, 2004].

Cohen WM, Florida R, Randazzese L, Walsh J. 1998. "Industry and the Academy: Uneasy Partners in the Cause of Technological Advance." In: Noll RG, ed. *Challenges to Research Universities*. Washington, DC: Brookings Institution Press. [On-line.] Available: brookings.nap.edu/books/0815715099/html/index.html [accessed July 28, 2004].

DeVol R, Wong P, Ki J, Bedroussian A, Koepp R. 2004. *America's Biotech and Life Science Clusters*. Santa Monica, CA: Milken Institute.

DHHS (Department of Health and Human Services). 1999. *Grants Policy Directive Part 3.02: Post-Award – Matching and Cost Sharing*. HHS Transmittal 99.05 (7/29/99).

Feller I. 1997. *Matching Fund and Cost-Sharing Experiences of U.S. Research Universities: Final Report to the National Science Foundation*. Bethesda, MD: COSMOS Corporation.

Feller I. 2000a. "Social Contracts and the Impact of Matching Fund Requirements on American Research Universities." *Educational Evaluation and Policy Analysis*, 22(Spring):91-98.

Feller I. 2000b. "The Remainder of the Cost Sharing Policy Agenda." *Research Management Review*, 11(Spring/Summer):31-39.

Hardy RB. 2000. "Cost Sharing—Past, Present—and Future?" *Research Management Review*, 11(Spring/Summer):9-19.

IOM (Institute of Medicine). 1997. *A Review of the Department of Defense's Program for Breast Cancer Research*. Washington, D.C.: National Academy Press.

Kettler HE. 2003. The Value of PPPs for Global Health (PowerPoint Presentation). Seattle, WA: Bill and Melinda Gates Foundation, October 27.

Kolker A. 2004. Presentation by Ann Kolker, Executive Director, Ovarian Cancer National Alliance, at the workshop held by the Committee on Alternative Funding Strategies for DOD's Peer Reviewed Medical Research Programs. National Academies, Washington, DC, April 26.

Larson EV, Brahmakulam IT. 2002. *Building a New Foundation for Innovation: Results of a Workshop for the National Science Foundation*. Santa Monica, CA: RAND. [On-line.] Available: www.rand.org/publications/MR/MR1534/index.html [accessed July 28, 2004].

NCI (National Cancer Institute). 2002. *A Public-Private Partnership between NCI and Avon*, reported by Michael Miller, October 1. [On-line.] Available: www.cancer.gov/templates/doc_bench.aspx?viewid=2eaa81ea-5d99-400d-9783-ad8eeb6f31b6&docid=b7096ffe-d020-4782-a9d8-d62454206571&print=1 [accessed July 13, 2004].

NCI-Avon. 2003. *Avon Foundation-NCI "Progress for Patients" Awards for Early Phase Clinical Interventions in Breast Cancer: Guidelines for Application, Review, and Award*. [On-line.] Available: www.cancer.gov/cancercenters/announcements/Avon2004.pdf [accessed July 28, 2004].

NRC (National Research Council). 2001. *The Advanced Technology Program: Assessing Outcomes*. Washington, DC: National Academies Press.

NSB (National Science Board). 1999. "National Science Foundation Statement on Cost Sharing." NSB-99-92. Arlington, VA: NSF. [On-line.] Available: www.nsf.gov/nsb/documents/archives.htm [accessed May 7, 2004].

NSB. 2002. *Science and Engineering Indicators – 2002*. NSB-02-1. Arlington, VA: National Science Foundation.

NSF (National Science Foundation). NSF. 2003a. Chapter X, "Management Challenges and Reforms," in *FY 2002 Performance and Accountability Report*. [On-line.] Available: www.nsf.gov/pubs/2003/nsf03023/pdf/chapter10.pdf [accessed May 7, 20004].

NSF. 2003b. Memorandum from Dr. Christine C. Boesz, Inspector General, NSF, to Dr. Warren Washington, Chair, National Science Board, and Dr. Rita R. Colwell, Director, NSF, "Management Challenges for NSF in 2004," October 17, 2003. [On-line.] Available: www.nsf.gov/pubs/2004/nsf0410/new_pdf/chapter4.pdf [accessed May 17, 2004].

NSF-OIG (National Science Foundation-Office of the Inspector General). 2002. *Semiannual Report to the Congress: March 2002*. [On-line.] Available: www.nsf.gov/pubs/2002/oigmarch2002/oigmarch2002.pdf [accessed May 7, 2004].

Seligman RP. 2000. "An Introduction to Cost Sharing: Why Good Deeds Do Not Go Unpunished." *Research Management Review*, 11(Spring/Summer):1-4.

University of California. 1996. *Trends in U.S. Funding for Biomedical Research*. San Francisco, CA: Center for the Health Professions and The Pew Scholars Program in the Biomedical Sciences, University of California, San Francisco. [On-line.] Available: www.futurehealth.ucsf.edu/pdf_files/usfunding.pdf [accessed July 28, 2004].

Visco F. 2004. Presentation by Fran Visco, President, National Breast Cancer Coalition, at the workshop held by the Committee on Alternative Funding Strategies for DOD's Peer Reviewed Medical Research Programs. National Academies, Washington, DC, April 26.

Widdus R. 2003. Private Sector Action for Health: Public-Private Partnerships (PowerPoint Presentation). Geneva: Initiative on Public-Private Partnerships for Health, July 23. [On-line.] Available: www.ippph.org/index.cfm?page=/ippph/publications&thechoice=retrieve&docno=55 [accessed July 28, 2004].

5

Findings and Recommendations

The Congressionally Directed Medical Research Programs (CDMRP) are a set of research funding initiatives on prevalent cancers and other diseases that have been administered by the U.S. Army Medical Research and Materiel Command (USAMRMC) of the Department of Defense (DOD) since 1992. The effort does not contribute directly to the principal medical mission of DOD, which is to prevent and treat war-related illnesses and wounds, but the work is relevant to the department's responsibility for the underlying health of military personnel and their dependents.

CDMRP is a small piece of the very large federal budget for national defense, which is under great strain because of current operations in Iraq and Afghanistan, as well as increased efforts to counter terrorism in other parts of the world. In response to a congressionally directed request by the DOD, the Institute of Medicine (IOM) formed a committee to report on the possibilities of augmenting the funding of CDMRP from nonfederal sources, identify mechanisms that could be used to leverage such funding, assess the impacts of alternative nonfederal sources and mechanisms of funding on CDMRP, and identify any legal or regulatory barriers to leveraging nonfederal funding. This committee did not formally evaluate the performance and results of CDMRP.

In forming its conclusions, the Committee on Alternative Funding Strategies for DOD's Peer Reviewed Medical Research Programs relied on the information gathered during the workshop, during conversations with CDMRP staff and stakeholders, and from the scientific literature addressing issues related to the funding of medical research. Because the literature on the benefits and costs of different research support mechanisms or the effects of leveraging of federal research and development (R&D) funding is sparse, this information was supplemented by committee members' judgment and experience as seekers of funding, recipients of governmental and private-sector research support, proposal reviewers, and managers of research programs.

This report addresses the question of whether it is possible and desirable to augment the appropriated dollars for CDMRP with funding from other sources. The answer to the of whether it is possible rests on an analysis of nonfederal sources of funding and mechanisms that may be available to access them, as well as potential impediments to that process. The answer to whether it is desirable rests on an analysis of how these other sources and funding mechanisms might affect the goals and effectiveness of CDMRP. Desirability also depends on how "augmentation" is defined. Augmentation of funding that increases public health, for example, by creating a critical mass of knowledge or skills, or by joining complementary resources that are needed to solve a problem, or by enabling results that would not otherwise be possible, is more desirable than augmentation that only serves to extend program funds, especially if the additional funds are not newly applied to biomedical research and are simply shifted from other biomedical research uses.

CDMRP occupies a niche in the spectrum of federally-funded medical research: it emphasizes high-risk exploratory research and new ideas by supporting projects that have little or no preliminary data and new investigators without an established track record in research. Based on testimony from program officials, grantees, and members of the advocacy community presented at an April 2004 workshop (see Appendix C for workshop agenda and participants) and an evaluation conducted by an earlier committee of the Institute of Medicine (IOM, 1997), the program appears to be well-run, supports high-quality research, and contributes to research progress in its areas of focus. It also concentrates its resources on research mechanisms that complement rather than duplicate the research approaches of the major funders of medical research in the United States, such as industry and the National Institutes of Health (NIH).

CDMRP's strategy of focusing on support of exploratory research, new investigators, and innovative approaches affects the prospects for outside funding. Funding of such work is generally and properly regarded as a function of the federal government, making up for market failures that result in private-sector underinvestment in these vital areas. Nonfederal funders—particularly philanthropic organizations and state governments—are unlikely sources. Given the disparity between the amount of federal resources relative to nonfederal resources, they have little motivation to provide funds unless they expect to leverage federal dollars for their priorities or they would like the federal program to pay for the application, peer review, and grants management processes.

Leveraging of nonfederal funds would happen most easily for certain types of research that are not the main focus of CDMRP and that are already supported by major funders of medical research. This includes later-stage research with applications that are likely to become commercially viable or possibly training or infrastructure grants. The possibility of co-funding from industry, the largest nonfederal funder of biomedical research, is least likely for early-stage exploratory research, which is one of the most important foci of CDMRP.

The committee concludes that CDMRP should pursue leveraging where it is appropriate, especially if it promises to leverage research results. Later-stage research initiatives, such as clinical research and clinical trials, are probably most appealing to other funders, although any initiative of possible interest to other funders might be pursued.

Leveraging would be facilitated if Congress granted the authority and means for the program to solicit and use outside funds for extramural awards. If private co-funding and other collaborations with CDMRP grow, there would have to be some changes in the way the program is currently run. For example, the potential risks inherent in public-private collaborations would need to be anticipated and addressed. Peer review of developmental research would need to involve a different set of experts than those who review exploratory research, for example, scientists who have successfully developed products and have some experience with identifying promising projects.

If CDMRP shifted emphasis from exploratory research to early-stage development of diagnostics; drugs, vaccines, and other therapeutics; and medical devices and other products, it would be in a better position to attract funds from venture capital and biotechnology and pharmaceutical companies. In accord with federal policy, however, this shift should be based on scientific grounds, not just to extend program funds. It should also consider the support that industry and other federal agencies already give to the development and testing of diagnostics, therapeutics, medical devices, and other efforts to develop commercial products and weigh that against the need for more high-risk/high-gain exploratory research to understand better the diseases addressed by CDMRP and identify potential points of intervention for preventing and treating them.

The committee was charged with assessing alternative nonfederal sources of support. It did not, therefore, consider some alternatives for leveraging CDMRP funds. For example, the committee did not assess how CDMRP might achieve greater progress in research by leveraging the resources of NIH and other federal biomedical research programs or by working out a more productive division of labor among the federal agencies that have similar program goals. The committee also did not look at the extent to which program rules and procedures could be revised to reduce the administrative burden on applicants and awardees and free additional time and other resources for research at applicant institutions—important issues that would need to be addressed elsewhere.

Recommendation 1: Facilitate Collaboration When Appropriate

Findings. The majority of funding of biomedical research comes from industry and is not readily accessible to a program such as CDMRP. Experience with cost sharing in other federal basic research programs shows that requiring recipients to provide significant percentages of the cost of projects to augment federal funds imposes additional expenses on both the recipient and the funder. This requirement also can have unintended—and often undesired—consequences (such as discouraging the submission of outstanding proposals from researchers at institutions with limited means) and may not substantially increase the total amount of funding in an area of research (or may redirect it from other important uses). Cost sharing is most appropriate when the co-funder receives a tangible benefit, and this is much more likely to happen in later-stage research or infrastructure projects rather than in basic and exploratory research. Yet CDMRP's greatest strength has been its support of new ideas and new investigators, where cost sharing beyond the provision of facilities and equipment is least justified.

The experience of federal R&D funding agencies with voluntary public-private collaborations generally has been positive, although collaborations must be individually negotiated, which can add significant costs to a project and increase the time it takes for the research to begin. Appendix A includes a number of examples in which foundations, companies, and state governments have partnered with federal agencies to fund a research project or program. In some cases, the nonfederal supporters of research have contributed dollars to the federal agency to use in funding research grants. In other cases, the nonfederal funding is not commingled with federal funds per se but is instead coordinated with them. For example, the federal and nonfederal collaborators fund different parts of an overall program or the nonfederal organization provides supplementary funding to a federal recipient. In some cases, a foundation or voluntary health agency funds applications that fall just below the pay line for federal grant programs, which saves them the costs of soliciting and reviewing proposals.

> **Recommendation 1. CDMRP should facilitate collaborative arrangements for funding research when collaboration would be beneficial and appropriate—for example, when it would achieve greater results through synergy or economies of scale or critical mass—but CDMRP should not expect such arrangements to augment significantly overall program funding.**

Opportunities for collaboration with other sponsors of biomedical R&D should be encouraged, not to stretch program funds, but to achieve program goals that could not be met otherwise. For example, increased funding might allow attainment of a critical mass in an area that no single funder could achieve, the development of a shared infrastructure, or the creation of a synergistic effect through the interactions of the different collaborators. In some cases, solving a particular problem may require interdependent inputs from more than one entity. Such collaborations generally will be targeted and time-limited, although they may be repeated or continued when each participant perceives it to be beneficial.

CDMRP should experiment with award mechanisms that facilitate collaborative R&D arrangements among academic institutions, industry, philanthropies, state governments, and/or other supporters of research, as has been done in the Breast Cancer Research Program with Collaborative-Clinical Translational Research Awards and Biotechnology Clinical Partnerships. These awards require collaborations to perform clinical trials, in the first case, between community-based oncology practices, the private sector, and academic centers, and in the second case, between a biotechnology company and an academic institution or health care organization. In addition, CDMRP should, through its inclusive planning process, develop programs that outside funders would be willing to help fund (see Recommendation 2, below). An alternative would be for CDMRP to approach nonfederal funders to explore the possibility that they might fund projects that receive high scores but that cannot be funded by CDMRP. This reliance on the CDMRP application and review process would save the nonfederal funders administrative costs.

Recommendation 2: Provide DOD with Gift Authority

Finding. Some federal agencies, such as NIH and the Centers for Disease Control and Prevention (CDC), have the authority to accept gifts for specified purposes and have foundations that can solicit private funds for their programs. Under current law and regulations, however, the Army is only allowed to accept private donations in its Army General Gift Fund for certain purposes (e.g., to benefit a school, hospital, library, museum, cemetery, or similar Army institution or organization), which do not include augmenting the funding of an extramural grant program such as CDMRP. Unlike some of these other federal research agencies, neither CDMRP nor its parent organization, USAMRMC, has the authority to receive outside funds to augment its budget for extramural awards. Even if it had such authority, it could not be used actively, as it is not legal for federal employees to seek funds from private sources.

The Henry M. Jackson Foundation for the Advancement of Military Medicine was established to be the recipient of funding for medical research and education projects from other federal and nonfederal sources, but only on behalf of the faculty of the Uniformed Services University of the Health Sciences, researchers at Walter Reed Army Institute of Research, and other intramural DOD researchers. The Jackson Foundation does not fund extramural research. Nonfederal funders also may contribute funds to the Defense Cooperation Account (DCA), but Congress must appropriate these funds and authorize their use for a specific purpose, and donors are asked not to designate the intended use of their contributions to DCA. If Congress wishes CDMRP to draw on foundations and private donors, it needs to provide the authority to receive gifts to support research administered by CDMRP or in collaboration with CDMRP.

Recommendation 2. Congress should provide the CDMRP with authority to:

a. receive gifts and donations from individuals, companies, foundations, and other organizations for the support of research grants and contracts awarded by CDMRP, and
b. charter a nonprofit foundation with authority to solicit and transfer nonfederal funds for the support of research grants and contracts awarded by CDMRP.

Gift authority might be granted to the Secretary of Defense, the Service Secretaries, or the Commander of USAMRMC, as long as it is delegated to the CDMRP program. A nonprofit foundation with the mission of assisting CDMRP or USAMRMC could be modeled after the Foundation for the National Institutes of Health or the CDC Foundation. Alternatively, the mission of the Henry M. Jackson Foundation could be expanded to include fundraising for CDMRP or USAMRMC extramural research programs. Based on the experience of similar foundations for other agencies, however, expectations of substantial donations to such a foundation should be modest. Congress also would have to provide for the additional costs of establishing and maintaining the foundation.

Recommendation 3: Limit Cost-Sharing/Matching Requirements

Finding. Cost-sharing and matching requirements do not always advance research goals. Usually, cost-shared funds do not expand the total funding provided for research. Rather, they involve the rechanneling of existing funding streams. In addition, cost-sharing requirements can impose additional administrative costs on both recipients and funders. Recipients must spend time seeking these sharing funds (or divert their own dollars from other uses), managing the relationships with donors, and documenting that the cost sharing was obtained and used properly. Funding agencies must ensure that the cost sharing was actually provided by all partners. Cost-sharing requirements thus generate additional administrative costs for all concerned. However, cost sharing makes sense where the extra costs are more than offset by additional benefits resulting from the partnership, such as when research results have foreseeable commercial applications.

Recommendation 3. CDMRP should not impose cost-sharing or matching fund requirements beyond those currently required, except when a tangible benefit to the award recipient is anticipated beyond the immediate term or scope of CDMRP-supported activity (for example, funding of instruments and facilities).

Care should be taken to see that cost sharing does not divert funds from other desirable activities, such as other research projects that would have been funded by those dollars. CDMRP should not let expectations of increased nonfederal funding shift the program's scientific priorities away from its focus on innovative exploratory research, research into disease prevention and causation, and epidemiological studies.

Recommendation 4: Issue Guidelines for Collaboration

Finding. Research on university-industry and government-industry partnerships and similar collaborations has identified a number of potential benefits and costs that result from these relationships. The benefits generally take the form of induced private investment in developing research results into commercial goods and services, but these benefits do not necessarily require co-funding or formal matching requirements. The costs can include the imposition of secrecy on the scientific process, the occurrence of delays and bias in the reporting of research results, the shifting of research priorities toward near-term development rather than long-term research, and the possibility of financial conflicts of interest for both research institutions and individual researchers.

Although collaborations with outside funders would be a useful adjunct to CDMRP efforts, their benefits should outweigh the additional costs involved, and the primacy of scientific excellence and program relevance can and should be maintained. Any pressure to shift program priorities away from basic exploratory research in order to maximize outside funding should be resisted. CDMRP policies and procedures regarding the protection of human subjects in research and avoidance of conflicts of interest should, of course, be rigorously applied.

> **Recommendation 4. DOD should issue guidelines for collaboration with the private sector, paying special attention to the potential impact of research collaborations with nonfederal funders on (a) program costs; (b) the integrity of the peer review process; (c) program priorities; (d) perceived and actual conflicts of interest; (e) openness in scientific communication; and (f) other issues that may arise in federal-private co-funding arrangements.**

Other research funding agencies have issued guidelines governing public-private collaborations, which could serve as models for DOD guidelines. The guidelines of NIH and CDC were described in Chapter 4. They focus on such issues as potential conflicts of interest that must be identified and addressed; intellectual property rights; the timely publication of research results; and the maintenance of academic freedom, and they contain suggestions of ways for avoiding or managing them.

REFERENCE

IOM (Institute of Medicine). 1997. *A Review of the Department of Defense's Program for Breast Cancer Research*. Washington, DC: National Academy Press.

A

Selected Federal Programs with Nonfederal Funding Participation[1]

DEPARTMENT OF DEFENSE (DOD)

Dual Use Science and Technology (DUS&T) Program

www.dtic.mil/dust/index.htm

DUS&T is a program with high visibility with Congress that generates applied or advanced technology projects through the creation and/or development of new products or process technologies that benefit the military. The applicant must be a for-profit company or have at least one for-profit firm on its team, and it must bear at least 50 percent of the cost of the effort (required by the fiscal year [FY] 1998 Defense Authorization Act), of which at least half must be "high quality"—that is, cash, labor or consumable materials. DOD funding contributions for approved projects are 25 percent from the Office of Undersecretary of Defense, and 25 percent from the service organization proposing the topic. Funding for the program was $40 million in FY 2002 (financed by a tax on all 6.1–6.3 research funds), $15.9 million in FY 2003, and $14.2 million in FY 2004; the request for FY 2005 is $5.2 million.

[1]Please note that the descriptions of these examples of collaborative funding of research are based on and often quoted directly from the websites that are cited in each case.

Government/Industry Co-sponsorship of University Research (GICUR) Program

www.acq.osd.mil/ddre/research/getinvolved.html

GICUR fosters cooperative, long-term basic research by universities with industry and/or government laboratories in research areas vital to the advancement of technologies important to DOD. Industry and government share responsibility for research area selection and overall direction as well as funding. For example, in cooperation with the Microelectronics Advanced Research Corporation (MARCO), the Semiconductor Electronics Microelectronics project funds four universities (University of California [UC] at Berkeley, Georgia Institute of Technology, Massachusetts Institute of Technology, and Carnegie Mellon) that in turn lead coordinated research efforts on particular topics by consortias of institutions. Under MARCO, the electronics industry provides at least three dollars for each dollar provided by DOD. Federal funding has averaged approximately $7 million a year since FY 1998.

Technology Investment Agreements (TIAs)

www.acq.osd.mil/dpap/Docs/RandD%20Text.doc

TIAs, authorized by 10 U.S.C. 2371, enable DOD to enter into research agreements other than grants and cooperative agreements. They permit the government to exercise greater flexibility and judgment to achieve program goals because they are not subject to many of the regulatory requirements (most notably, the Baye-Dole Act patent provision) of standard federal grants and cooperative agreements that deter some companies from partnering with the government. Cost sharing of at least half of the project costs is required, however. According to DODs Grant and Agreement Regulations (section 37.215), "The purpose of cost share is to ensure that the recipient incurs real risk that gives it a vested interest in theproject's success." TIAs also require "a greater level of involvement of the government program officials in the execution of the research than the usual oversight of a research grant or procurement contract."

Twenty-eight TIAs and cooperative agreements were entered into in FY 2001, with industry paying for 46 percent of the total costs of $114 million (www.acq.osd.mil/dpap/Docs/FY01RPT.doc). For example, in 2000 DARPA entered into a TIA with Motorola, Inc. for an 18-month effort to develop a multichip module sample preparation system for genetic analysis. DOD wanted access to Motorola's technology, but Motorola does not accept standard government research contracts. Use of the TIA permitted the company to use its existing accounting systems, which were not compliant with FAR, and to negotiate other rights important to Motorola, including alternate disputes resolution procedures, intellectual property rights less stringent than the Bayh-Dole provision, and foreign access to technology. In return, Motorola paid for $1.5 million of the $4.9 million cost of the project.

Thin-Film Photovoltaics Partnerships Program

www.nrel.gov/business_opportunities/pdfs/4_44205_loi.pdf

The Thin-Film Photovoltaics Partnerships Program is a competitive grant program intended to accelerate the progress of thin film solar cells and module development as well as to address mid- and long-term research and development issues. Cost sharing of up to 50 percent is expected from industry, depending on size of company and type of participation. Cost sharing must be all cash; in-kind is not accepted. The applicant's level of cost sharing is a factor in the cost evaluation of proposals, in addition to technical merit. No cost sharing is required from academic institutions.

Technologies for Metabolic Monitoring and Julia Weaver Fund Research Program

www.momrp.org/tmm.jsp

The Technologies for Metabolic Monitoring (TMM) and Julia Weaver Fund (JWF) Research Program is a collaborative initiative between the U.S. Army Medical Research and Materiel Command, Juvenile Diabetes Research Foundation (JDRF), NASA, and the National Institute of Diabetes and Digestive and Kidney Diseases (NIDDK). Its goal is to unite metabolic monitoring technologies for the military and civilians, align these with the needs of the two populations, and ultimately improve the quality and range of metabolic monitoring technologies available to all. Funding focuses on supporting and assisting in the identification and maturation of potential new, novel, and innovative technologies and techniques for the monitoring and assessment of metabolism, especially those that may apply to the care and long-term health maintenance of diabetic patients. The collaborating entities participate in an advisory group for the research program.

TMM/JWF is congressionally supported and secured a total of $9.3 million in federal appropriations through FY 2003. The FY 2004 program announcement anticipated a total of $3 million in awards

DEPARTMENT OF ENERGY (DOE)

Fusion Science Centers

www.sc.doe.gov/grants/Fr03-26.html

In 2003, the Office of Fusion Energy Sciences in DOE's Office of Science issued a notice inviting grant applications for fusion science centers that focus on fundamental issues in fusion plasma science. The University of Maryland/University of California at Los Angeles and the University of Rochester were selected to host the centers in May, 2004. The duration of the grants is five years and may be renewed once for another five years. Total funding for the two centers over the initial five-year grant is expected to be nearly $12 million. The host institution is required to provide at least 15 percent matching funds for the center.

NATIONAL AERONAUTICS AND SPACE ADMINISTRATION (NASA)

Research Partnership Centers

spd.nasa.gov/research_centers.html

The Space Partnership Development (SPD) Office, part of NASA's Office of Biological and Physical Research, exists to enable industry to conduct research and develop products on the International Space Station (ISS) and other NASA space and ground missions. One component of the SPD is a program with 15 research partnership centers, each working with companies, universities, and other organizations in a specific field of research. Each center is a consortium of academia, government, and industry partnering to develop new or improved services and products, usually through collaborative research conducted in outer space. NASA provides an annual base grant and the centers receive cash and in-kind contributions from industry, universities, research institutions, and other governmental agencies (federal, state, and local). In FY 2002, the ratio of non-NASA to SPD funding was 2.15:1. The centers received $33.1 million from industry and $30.6 million from other sources, with $29.6 million from SPD and $4.3 million from other NASA centers. Of the total of $63.7 million in nonfederal funding, $33.0 million was cash and the rest was in-kind.

NATIONAL INSTITUTES OF HEALTH (NIH)

Academic Public Private Partnership Program (AP4)

dtp.nci.nih.gov/docs/ap4/handbook/index.html

Modeled after the Industry/University Cooperative Research Center Program of the National Science Foundation, AP4 is a partnership initiative whose goal is to conduct novel cancer therapeutic, prevention, diagnostic, and imaging research to hasten the translation of research findings into clinical trials. The research occurs at an academic center with the advice and support of industry, nonprofit institutes, government partners, and the National Cancer Institute (NCI). Formed by NCI through its Developmental Therapeutics Program in the Division of Cancer Treatment and Diagnosis, the effort was initiated in July 2003 through the mechanism of inviting applications for one-year planning grants. Planning grant applicants are expected to utilize the funds to study the feasibility of developing the pharmaceutical/non-profit/academic interactions necessary to establish and support an AP4 Center, and to actually prepare the application. NCI intends to use approximately $1.124 million in FY 2004 appropriations to fund up to 15 planning grants.

Alzheimer's Disease Neuroimaging Initiative (ADNI)
grants.nih.gov/grants/guide/rfa-files/RFA-AG-04-005.html
www.fnih.org/images/Prelim2003ar.pdf

This public-private partnership initiative will develop a multisite, longitudinal, prospective, naturalistic study of normal cognitive aging, mild cognitive impairment, and early Alzheimer's disease as a public domain research resource. A primary goal of ADNI is to identify the biomarkers of disease progression that are most promising for use as surrogate endpoints in clinical trials. ADNI was established by an RFA issued by the National Institute on Aging (NIA) in October 2003. Other partners involved in the consortium include academic investigators, the Food and Drug Administration, the Alzheimer's Association, the Institute for the Study of Aging, and participating pharmaceutical and medical imaging companies.

The companies that contribute funds will be on the steering committee for the project, but they will not have special privileges, such as early access to the data. The clinical, imaging, and biological data will be made available, with appropriate safeguards to ensure participant privacy, to all scientific investigators in the academic and industrial research communities. Biological samples of blood and cerebrospinal fluid will be equitably distributed to qualified scientists, based on the quality and significance of proposed studies for them. Cell lines will also be established for distribution to qualified scientists.

One U01 cooperative agreement award will be made to the successful applicant, which will support the other parts of ADNI—including the coordinating center, the neuroimaging center, and the clinical sites—through subcontracts. The plan is to spend $60 million on the initiative over five years, with approximately $40 million coming from NIA and $20 million from pharmaceutical and medical imaging companies. Private-sector funding for the initiative is arranged through the Foundation for the NIH (FNIH) (because NIH staff cannot solicit funds from private companies), which will accept monies and transfer them to the institute to help pay for the program. Eli Lilly and Company has pledged $2.5 million over five years and FNIH is discussing pledges with additional companies.

Animal Models of Diabetic Complications Consortium
www.amdcc.org

Established in late 2001, the intent of this initiative is to assemble a cross-disciplinary consortium to develop innovative animal models that closely mimic the human complications of diabetes. The consortium will consist of eight mouse engineering and phenotyping units from different institutions and a coordinating and bioinformatics unit. The administrative and funding instrument to be used for this program will be a cooperative agreement as set out in an RFA involving the National Institute of Diabetes and Digestive and Kidney Diseases, the National Heart, Lung, and Blood Institute (NHLBI), the National Eye Institute, the National Institute of Dental and Craniofacial Research (NIDCR), and the JDRF. NIH intended to commit approximately $4.5 million in FY 2001 to fund up to five or six of the former and to fund the latter as well. JDRF intended to commit up to $500,000 to this program.

Best Pharmaceuticals for Children

www.fda.gov/opacom/laws/pharmkids/contents.html

The Best Pharmaceuticals for Children Act of 2002 called for FNIH (www.fnih.org/aboutus/board.shtml) to raise funds to enable testing of drugs that are approved for adult use and used off-label to treat children but have not been tested for treatment of children for safety and efficacy. The public-private collaborative subsequently created is headed by a 15-member advisory committee representing patient groups and the American Academy of Pediatrics. Contributors include AstraZeneca LP, Aventis Pharmaceuticals Inc., Boehringer Ingelheim Cares Foundation, Inc., Dr. and Mrs. Samuel E. Broder, Eli Lilly and Company Foundation, Novartis Pharmaceuticals Corporation, Pfizer Inc., Merck Company Foundation, and Wyeth. Merck made the first contribution of $1 million over three years, and pledges totaled $3.6 million at the end of 2003 (www.fnih.org/images/Prelim2003ar.pdf).

Cooperative Research Program for Improved Hemophilia Therapy

www.nhlbi.nih.gov/funding/fromdir/cong/cj.htm

The FY 2005 NHLBI budget indicates that the Institute and the National Hemophilia Foundation are planning a cooperative research program to improve treatments for bleeding disorders such as hemophilia or von Willebrand disease. The program was in the proposal stage at the time that this report was completed and no further details concerning it were available.

Endocrine Pancreas Consortium

www.cbil.upenn.edu/EPConDB/

The public-private Endocrine Pancreas Consortium originally sought to identify all genes expressed in the developing endocrine pancreas and to generate both microarray and bioinformatics tools, which could be used to study development, function, and disease progression in type 1 diabetes. A supplemental objective was added in FY 2001 to screen cDNA libraries for clones that might be useful as markers for beta cell precursors. NIDDK and the Juvenile Diabetes

Research Foundation International (JDRF) awarded two resource-related grants in FY 1999 to the Washington University Genome Sequencing Center and the University of Pennsylvania Center for Bioinformatics to establish the consortium. A database (EPConDB) and tools to query sequence and expression data generated have been created under the aegis of the Beta Cell Biology Consortium (www.betacell.org/).

The Etiology, Pathogenesis and Treatment of ALS
grants.nih.gov/grants/guide/rfa-files/RFA-NS-04-003.html

This public/private partnership was formed to solicit applications to support research in the causes, pathobiology of motor neurons and associated cell types, and the diagnosis and treatment of amyotrophic lateral sclerosis (ALS). The National Institute of Neurological Disorders and Stroke (NINDS), the Department of Veterans Affairs (VA), and the ALS Association intend to commit a total of approximately $2.4 million in FY 2004 to fund approximately 10 new grants in response to this RFA. An applicant may request a project period of up to 2 years and a budget for direct costs of up to $275,000 over the course of two years for NIH awards, or a budget for direct costs of up to $500,000 over the course of two years for VA awards.

Gene Therapy Approaches for Cystic Fibrosis and Other Heart, Lung, and Blood Diseases
grants.nih.gov/grants/guide/rfa-files/RFA-HL-93-008.html

This public-private program encourages innovative, high-risk gene therapy directions by new or established investigators through pilot/feasibility studies. Established in 1992 by NHLBI and the Cystic Fibrosis Foundation (CFF), NHLBI issued an RFA for program project grants for research on gene therapy approaches to cystic fibrosis (CF) and other heart, lung, and blood disease. Applicants could request up to $1.33 million in total costs for the first year. Up to $250,000 of the $1.33 million could be used to fund non-CF -related pilot/feasibility studies. For CF-related pilot/feasibility studies, CFF indicated it would provide each grantee up to $500,000 per year in additional funds in direct costs per year.

Gene Therapy Core Centers
grants.nih.gov/grants/guide/rfa-files/RFA-DK-97-010.html

This public-private initiative invites applications for core center grants to support gene therapy research on cystic fibrosis and other genetic diseases of interest to NIDDK. Cosponsored in 1992 by NIDDK and CFF, in FY 1993 NIDDK awarded two five-year grants on a competitive basis, using the core (P30) grant mechanism. In FY 1998 and FY 1999, NIDDK continued the initial two centers and funded a new center. In each case, through separate awards, CFF awarded the centers up to $500,000 per year in direct costs for 5 years for pilot and feasibility studies to develop gene therapy for cystic fibrosis. To be eligible for CFF funding, applicants had to provide the CFF with a copy of the NIDDK review. In the 2004 recompetition, NIDDK assumed funding for pilot and feasibility studies. The three existing centers were refunded, a fourth center was added, and their name was changed to Molecular Therapy Core Centers.

Global Network for Women's and Children's Health Research

gn.rti.org

The Global Network for Women's and Children's Health Research is a collaborative effort to create an international research network to improve the health of women and children throughout the world. It was formed by the National Institute of Child Health and Human Development (NICHHD) and several other NIH institutes (National Institute of Allergy and Infectious Diseases [NIAID], National Cancer Institute, NIDCR, National Institute of Mental Health (NIMH), National Center for Complementary and Alternative Medicine), the Fogarty International Center, and the Bill and Melinda Gates Foundation. The network was initiated in 2001 with $15 million each from the Gates Foundation and NICHD. The other institutes are providing financial, technical, scientific, training, and administrative support. The first eight scientific team units, consisting of a U.S. principal investigator and a senior scientist in a developing country, were funded in 2003, with each receiving approximately $500,000 per year over five years. In addition, there is funding for a data coordinating center at RTI International and for special projects.

Grants for Research on the Effects of Hypoglycemia on Neuronal and Glial Cell Function

grants.nih.gov/grants/guide/rfa-files/RFA-NS-02-008.html

This public-private initiative focuses on elucidating the effects of acute and recurrent episodes of hypoglycemia on glial and neuronal cells of the developing and mature central nervous system. The National Institute of Neurological Disorders and Stroke (NINDS), the NIDDK, and the JDRF funded six grants in September 2002 intended to enhance understanding of the effects of hypoglycemia on brain function and lead to new targets for therapeutic intervention of this serious complication. According to the RFA for this initiative, NINDS and NIDDK intended to commit approximately $1.25 million in FY 2002. JDRF intended to commit up to $250,000 in additional funds to cofund research project grants that are both scientifically meritorious and fit within the JDRF mission and research emphasis areas.

Grants for Research on Innovative Approaches to Disease Prevention through Behavior Change

grants.nih.gov/grants/guide/rfa-files/RFA-OD-98-002.html
www.od.nih.gov/behaviorchange/index.htm

In 1997, a large number of NIH components (12 institutes and 5 offices) and the American Heart Association (AHA) cosponsored an RFA inviting applications for a four-year research grant program to test interventions designed to achieve long-term health behavior change. AHA sponsored semi-annual grantee workshops associated with the RFA. The sponsoring organizations committed approximately $8 million annually from FY 1999 to FY 2002 to fund 15 research grants selected on the basis of the scientific review. A Behavioral Change Consortium comprised of NIH program staff, research investigators at the individual sites, and representatives from co-sponsoring private foundations was established to explore the opportunities for further collaboration across the studies. In 2003, a summary report of the research effort was released (www.od.nih.gov/behaviorchange/summary/summary.htm).

Immune Tolerance Network (ITN)

www.immunetolerance.org/

ITN is a consortium of approximately 80 basic and clinical scientists and physicians at more than 40 institutions in the United States, Canada, and Europe. Its purpose is to conduct basic and clinical trials on ways to improve the success of kidney transplants and pancreatic islet transplants by selectively disabling immune cells that attack transplanted tissues while allowing other immune cells to function normally and to induce tolerance in autoimmune diseases, asthma, and allergy. ITN was established in 1999 by NIAID, NIDDK, and JDRF. ITN is headquartered at the UC San Francisco and is funded by a joint contract from NIH and JDRF. The initiative was funded for $144 million over 7 years, with $130 million from NIH and $14 million from JDRF. JDRF also provides discretionary funding directly to ITN to finance research-related activities that cannot be supported with federal funding.

Innovative Research on Human Mucosal Immunity

grants.nih.gov/grants/guide/rfa-files/RFA-AI-99-011.html

This public-private initiative offered exploratory/developmental research grants to attract new investigators and support novel research into understanding the human mucosal immune system. Cofunded by NIAID and the National Institute of Dental and Craniofacial Research (NIDCR) and the Crohn's and Colitis Foundation of America, approximately 15 grants in FY 2000 totaling $3.1 million were to be awarded.

International Type 1 Diabetes Genetics Consortium (T1DGC)
www.t1dgc.org/

T1DGC is an international collaborative (with Asia-Pacific, European, North American, and United Kingdom networks) to facilitate the genetic analysis of Type 1 diabetes via the sharing of reagents, methods, strategies, samples, knowledge, and data at all levels of the research effort. A joint initiative of NIH and JDRF, the consortium will transmit collected DNA samples to the Center for Inherited Disease Research for whole-genome scan analysis, provide resources for genetic analyses to the scientific community, and deposit samples, at least initially, in a regional network repository. Recruitment has started in the four regional networks. JDRF provided the organizational funding, supplies complementary funding when needed, and is an ongoing participant in consortium agenda and decisions.

Islet Cell Resource (ICR) Centers
icr.coh.org/

Ten regional ICR centers were established in September 2001 to both provide clinical grade human islets to investigators engaged in islet transplantation protocols throughout the country and optimize the procedures used to obtain such islets. The ICR initiative was developed by the National Center for Research Resources (NCRR), NIDDK, and JDRF. In addition to the centers, NCRR is supporting an administrative and bioinformatics coordinating center (ABCC). Over their five-year duration, the awards made to these centers should reach a total of up to $11million in direct costs, plus $3.5 million to the ABCC to support the ICR infrastructure. NIDDK and JDRF are providing additional financial support based on the number of islet cell preparations made annually by each of the awardees. A representative of JDRF serves on the ICR sterring committee.

Mouse Sequencing Consortium (MSC)
www.genome.gov/10002191

Formed in October 2000, MSC was a public-private partnership coordinated by FNIH. This program was established to speed up the determination of the DNA sequence of the mouse genome and make the information available to the public quickly and without restrictions. Six NIH institutes (NCI, National Human Genome Research Institute, National Institute on Deafness and Other Communication Disorders, NIDDK, NINDS, NIMH) provided funding in the amount of $34 million; Wellcome Trust, $7.75 million; SmithKline Beecham, $6.5 million; Merck Genome Research Institute, $6.5 million; and Affymetrix, Inc. $3.5 million; for a total of approximately $58 million. The funding principally supported work at three DNA sequencing laboratories: the Whitehead Institute for Biomedical Research in Cambridge, MA, the Washington University School of Medicine in St. Louis, MO, and the Sanger Centre in the United Kingdom. The project's goal of generating three-fold coverage of the mouse DNA sequence in six months, representing at least 95 percent of the full complement of mouse DNA, was achieved (www.nhgri.nih.gov/10002158). The effort was continued and broadened, and the international Mouse Genome Sequencing Consortium published a high-quality draft sequence of the mouse genome and a comparative analysis of the mouse and human genomes in the December 5, 2002, issue of *Nature*.

Multilateral Initiative on Malaria (MIM)

www.who.int/tdr/diseases/malaria/mim.htm

Founded in 1997, is an international collaboration in scientific research against malaria. MIM's U.S. governmental supporters include NIH's Fogarty International Center, National Library of Medicine, and NIAID. FNIH is the fiscal agent, collecting and distributing funds that enable the initiative to develop training programs. During the period 2000-2002, FNIH received funding from GlaxoSmithKline, the Gates Foundation, the Ellison Foundation, Burroughs Wellcome Fund, Wellcome Trust, the Rockefeller Foundation, the United Nations Foundation, and the World Bank. The governments of Norway, Sweden, The Netherlands, Demark, the United Kingdom, Germany, and Canada have also provided significant funding.

Senator Paul D. Wellstone Muscular Dystrophy Cooperative Research Centers

www.niams.nih.gov/rtac/funding/grants/muscular_dystrophy_2004.htm

The NIH Muscular Dystrophy Cooperative Research Center (MDCRC) Program was established in October 2003 as a public-private collaboration among the National Institute of Arthritis and Musculoskeletal and Skin Diseases (NIAMS), the National Institute of Neurological Disorders and Stroke, the National Institute of Child Health and Human Development, and the Muscular Dystrophy Association (MDA) to fund three extramural centers (University of Pittsburgh, University of Washington, and University of Rochester) for research on the muscular dystrophies, a group of genetic diseases that result in muscle weakness and wasting. The institutes will fund the three centers (selected through competitive peer review) at $1 million a year each in direct costs for five years. MDA will provide up to $500,000 in supplemental funding per center per year for three years. A 2004 RFA anticipates funding of up to three additional centers in FY 2005. The program was renamed in honor of Senator Paul Wellstone in 2004.

National Cancer Institute/Affymetrix Human Transcriptome Project (HTP)

cgap.nci.nih.gov/Genes/Affy

Initiated in 2001, this project is a collaboration between the private-sector research firm Affymetrix and NCI to determine the gene expression profiles of normal, precancerous, and cancerous cells, leading eventually to improved detection, diagnosis, and treatment. As part of NCI's Cancer Genome Anatomy Project, HTP's goal is to generate the complete collection of transcribed elements of the human genome.

Neurobiology of Diabetic Complications

grants.nih.gov/grants/guide/rfa-files/RFA-NS-00-002.html

This public-private collaborative program supports research on the mechanisms by which diabetes results in painful, disabling peripheral neuropathy, autonomic neuropathy, impaired counter-regulation and hypoglycemia unawareness, and other neurological complications. In FY 2000, NINDS, NIDDK, and JDRF awarded 18 two- to four-year grants on diabetic neuropathy. The NIH institutes managed the review and the JDRF suggested reviewers, encouraged applications and provided part of the funding. These were awarded under two initiatives supported by special statutory funds for type 1 diabetes (RFA-NS-99-005 and RFA-NS-00-002).

NIH Challenge Grants and Partnerships Program

The FY 2000 Public Health and Social Services Emergency Fund appropriation included $20 million for an NIH Challenge Grants and Partnership Program. The purpose of the legislation was to promote joint ventures between NIH and the biotechnology, pharmaceutical, and medical device industries. One-on-one matching of federal dollars by qualified organizations that are conducting R&D activities in biomedical research or biotechnology with commercial potential or conducting research in promising therapies was required.

Partnerships: Hepatitis B and Vector Borne Diseases Control

grants.nih.gov/grants/guide/rfa-files/RFA-AI-03-003.html

In this partnership initiative, NIAID uses the U01 cooperative agreement funding mechanism to develop and test products for certain infectious diseases. A key component of this initiative is the development of productive partnerships between the federal government, universities, and the biotechnology, chemical, and/or pharmaceutical industries. All projects must demonstrate the substantive involvement of a for-profit company, defined as the commitment of one or more of resources such as funds, personnel, or in-kind contributions of materials and/or reagents, data management resources, or regulatory support. Industry invests little in the commercialization of products to control a number of infectious diseases of great public health importance because it foresees little profit. This initiative is aimed at stimulating industry to participate by providing funding that reduces investment risks for companies, for example, providing critical decision-making data for industry through support of antimicrobial screening; formulation, toxicology, and pharmacokinetics; regulatory filing; and clinical trials.

Partnerships for Vaccine and Diagnostic Development
grants.nih.gov/grants/guide/rfa-files/RFA-AI-03-028.html

This initiative is basically the same as the Hepatitis B and Vector Borne Diseases Control partnership initiative except it is focused on the development of vaccines against and diagnostics for group A streptococci and group B streptococci and vaccines against *Helicobacter pylori.* Substantial involvement of industry is also required in this program.

Challenge Grants: Biodefense Product Development
grants.nih.gov/grants/guide/rfa-files/RFA-AI-04-029.html

This NIAID public-private initiative was established in 2004 to support further development of previously identified products against NIAID Category A, B, and C priority pathogens, including vaccines, adjuvants, therapeutics, and diagnostics. Under this program, partnerships among government, industry, academic institutions, and non-profit research organizations are encouraged. All projects must demonstrate substantive investment by industry participants, including funding, personnel, and in-kind contributions of materials, reagents, or other resources. With an anticipated July 2005 award date, this RFA will use the mechanism of the NIH challenge grant-cooperative agreement, and the applicant will be solely responsible for planning, directing, and executing the proposed project. The approximately four to eight awards will be made for a period of up to three years and will be performance based. The estimated total funds (direct and facilities and administrative costs) available for all awards for the duration of the program will be $30 million.

Osteoarthritis Initiative Public-Private Consortium

www.niams.nih.gov/ne/oi/index.htm

The Osteoarthritis Initiative (OAI) is a $60 million collaborative consortium between NIH and pharmaceutical companies to pool funds and expertise to create a public repository of osteoarthritis patient data, radiological information, and biological specimens. OAI is coordinated from the public sector by the NIAMS and NIA, with additional support from six other NIH institutes and centers. The private-sector partners are Merck, Novartis Pharmaceuticals Corporation, and Pfizer. Four clinical centers (University of Maryland School of Medicine, Ohio State University, University of Pittsburgh, and Memorial Hospital of Rhode Island), and a data coordinating center (UC San Francisco) were chosen in July 2002 from competitively reviewed applications submitted in response to Requests for Proposals. All partners have agreed that clinical data and x-ray information will be freely accessible to qualified scientists everywhere. For other resources that are limited (such as biological specimens), priority will be given to researchers studying promising biomarkers that will be made widely available for research and commercial use. The private-sector members of the consortium pool their resources, expected to total approximately $22 million, with NIH's appropriated funds through FNIH. In addition, Siemens Medical is collaborating with the OAI by enabling the NIH discounted purchases of the 3T field-strength magnets for each of the clinical centers and working with NIH to insure the highest performance of these systems.

Overcoming Barriers to Early Phase Clinical Trials Initiative

www.focr.org/programs/publicprivate.htm
www.fnih.org/partners/translational_research/overcomingbarriers.shtml

In this public-private partnership, five industry partners (Aventis Pharmaceuticals Inc., Bristol-Myers Squibb, Eli Lilly and Company, GlaxoSmithKline, and Novartis Pharmaceuticals Corporation) and a private nonprofit group (Friends of Cancer Research) collaborate with the National Cancer Institute to reduce health disparities among underserved populations. Funds from the private sector partners are provided through FNIH. The initiative works to increase access to early phase clinical trials and to identify and overcome the barriers that prevent their participation. For example, six cancer centers chosen by an NIH peer review committee were awarded grants in August 2003 to design and implement new approaches to recruiting elderly and minority volunteers to clinical trials. The private sector partners contribute to this $5.7 million initiative through FNIH.

Pathogenesis and Treatment of Cystic Fibrosis

grants.nih.gov/grants/guide/rfa-files/RFA-DK-95-006.html

This public-private initiative involves grants to conduct basic research on the pathogenesis of cystic fibrosis and its complications, related applied cell and molecular biology, translational, and clinical research, and potential therapies. In 1995, NIDDK, NHLBI, and CFF cosponsored the RFA for this program. For FY 1996, $2 million in total costs were to be committed by NIDDK and $1 million by NHLBI to fund applications submitted in response to this RFA. An additional $2 million were to be committed by CFF to fund applications not funded by NIDDK or NHLBI. Approximately 15 awards were anticipated. The committee did not identify any information indicating whether and how the funds were distributed.

Training Programs in Diabetes Research for Pediatric Endocrinologists
grants.nih.gov/grants/guide/rfa-files/RFA-DK-02-024.html

This public-private initiative established joint programs for the research training and career development of pediatric endocrinologists to foster development of a diverse and highly trained workforce of pediatric endocrinologists able to lead research efforts in the area of pediatric diabetes. NIDDK, the American Diabetes Association (ADA), and JDRF awarded seven combined T32/K12 training program grants in FY 2002 and FY 2003, with NIDDK intending to commit approximately $1.5 million to the initiative in FY 2002.

Transitional Career Development Award in Women's Health Research
www.niams.nih.gov/rtac/funding/grants/rfa/od_00_003.pdf

This award is designed to support career development experiences leading to independence for clinical investigators interested in patient-oriented or population-based research related to women's health. Salary for the first two years is funded by Pfizer Women's Health of Pfizer, Inc. (through a grant to FNIH), allowing awardees to conduct clinical research in the NIH intramural program. This is followed by two years at an academic institution, funded by 12 NIH institutes and centers and the Office of Research on Women's Health (ORWH) through K22 Career Transition Awards.

Translational Research for the Prevention and Control of Diabetes
grants.nih.gov/grants/guide/pa-files/PA-02-153.html

In 2002, this initiative was established to solicit research to translate recent advances in the prevention and treatment of type 1 or type 2 diabetes into clinical practice for individuals and communities at risk. It was formed by several NIH institutes (NIDDK, the National Eye Institute [NEI], the National Institute of Nursing Research [NINR], the Office of Behavioral and Social Sciences Research, the Agency for Healthcare Research and Quality, the Centers for Disease Control and Prevention [CDC]), and ADA. An expansion of an earlier program announcement sponsored by NIDDK, NEI, NINR, and ADA (grants.nih.gov/grants/guide/pa-files/PA-01-069.html), this NIH research demonstration and dissemination project (R18) is the award mechanism used to fund this initiative. The R18 is designed to support the testing and evaluation of interventions and activities that lead to application of existing knowledge to disease control and prevention.

Triggers and Environmental Determinants of Diabetes in Youth (TEDDY)

www.niddk.nih.gov/patient/TEDDY/TEDDY.htm

TEDDY is a public-private consortium formed to identify newborns at high genetic risk and follow them for the development of type 1 diabetes, with a goal of organizing international efforts to identify infectious agents, dietary factors, or other environmental factors that trigger type 1 diabetes in genetically susceptible individuals. Several NIH institutes (NIDDK, NIAID, NICHD, the National Institute of Environmental Health Sciences [NIEHS]), CDC, ADA, and JDRF are the sponsors of this project. Seven cooperative agreements were signed in September 2002 for a data coordinating center and six clinical centers.

Type 1 Diabetes TrialNet

www.diabetestrialnet.org/en/index.html

TrialNet is a collaborative network of clinical centers, experts in diabetes and immunology, and specialized laboratories and other facilities. It was formed in September 2001 by NIDDK, NICHD, NIAID, JDRF, and ADA. It consists of 14 clinical centers in the United States and Canada funded by grants from NIDDK and the 4 international clinical centers (in Italy, Finland, the United Kingdom, and Australia) funded by JDRF. According to the RFA for this initiative (grants.nih.gov/grants/guide/notice-files/NOT-DK-01-006.html), approximately $4.8 million in total costs per year will be committed to provide personnel and supplies to the Clinical Centers in order to complete DPT-1 and initiate planning for future studies, with a cap of approximately $242,000 per clinical center per year in total costs.

Understanding Hypoglycemia Unawareness in Patients with Type 1 Diabetes

grants.nih.gov/grants/guide/rfa-files/RFA-DK-01-031.html

This public-private initiative fosters basic and clinical research on molecular mechanisms underlying hypoglycemia unawareness and novel approaches to prevent or reverse this condition in diabetic patients. In September 2002, NIDDK, NINDS, NICHD, NINR, and JDRF awarded eight research grants relevant to hypoglycemia unawareness for funding periods of two to five years. The RFA for this initiative indicated that the NIH institutes intended to commit approximately $3.25 million in FY 2002 to fund four to eight grants, and that JDRF intended to commit up to $500,000 in additional funds to co-fund research project grants that are both scientifically meritorious and fit within their mission and research emphasis areas.

Other NIH Programs with Federal-Private Funding

Bioengineering for Disease Prevention and Control: National Center for Research Resources (NCRR) and the Whitaker Foundation (RFA-RR-94-005).

Cooperative Program on Retinal Degenerative Disease Research: NEI and the Foundation Fighting Blindness. Supports R01grants; R41, R42, R43, R44 small business grants; K08, K23, K24 career development awards (PA-00-009).

Cooperative Study Group for Autoimmune Disease Prevention: NIAID, NIDDK, NICHD, NIDCR, NIAMS, ORWH, and JDRF. Supports U19 multi-project cooperative agreements (RFA-AI-00-016).

Diabetes Centers of Excellence: NIDDK, NIAID, and JDRF. Funds P01 program project grants (RFA-DK-99-002).

Foodborne Illnesses, Gastrointestinal and Renal Complications: NIDDK and the American Digestive Health Foundation. Funds R01 and R21 grants (RFA-DK-00-008).

Health Care Access, Quality and Insurance for Low-Income Children: Agency for Health Care Policy and Research and the David and Lucile Packard Foundation. Supports U01 cooperative agreements (RFA-HS-99-005).

Helicobacter pylori *and its Relationship to Digestive Diseases and Cancer*: NIDDK, NCI, NIAID, Office of Research on Minority Health (ORMH), and the American Digestive Health Foundation. Supports R01 research project grants; R29 FIRST awards; R03 small grants (RFA-DK-97-003).

Hepatitis C: Natural History, Pathogenesis, Therapy and Prevention: NIDDK, NCI, NIAID, National Institute on Alcohol Abuse and Alcoholism, National Institute on Drug Abuse, Office of AIDS Research, ORMH, and the American Digestive Health Foundation. Funds R01 grants (RFA-DK-98-017).

Human Islet Transplantation into Humans: NIDDK, NIAID, and JDRF. Funds R01 grants and Interactive Research Project Grant awards (RFA-DK-99-006)

Indo-US Vaccine Action Program Starr Grants: Funds donated to the NIAID Restricted Gift Fund by the Starr Foundation. Supports supplements to current grants or R03 awards (NOT-99-097).

Integrative Approaches to the Study of Motility of the Gastrointestinal Tract: NIDDK, ORWH, and the American Digestive Health Foundation. Funds R01 and R21 grants (RFA-DK-99-004).

Mentored Clinical Scientist Awards in Nephrology: NIDDK and the National Kidney Foundation. Supports K08 clinical scientist development awards (PAR-98-064).

***Mouse Models of Diabetic Complications Consortium*:** NIDDK, NHLBI, NEI, NIDCR, and JDRF. Supports U01 cooperative agreements (RFA-DK-01-009).

***NINDS Administrative Supplements: FDA-Approved Compound Screens for Neurodegeneration*:** NINDS, Huntington's Disease Society of America, the ALS Association, and the Hereditary Diseases Foundation. (NOT-NS-01-009).

***Paul B. Beeson Career Development Awards in Aging*:** NIA, the John A. Hartford Foundation, the Atlantic Philanthropies, and the Starr Foundation. Supports K23 patient-oriented research career development awards and K08 mentored clinical scientist development awards (RFA-AG-05-001).

***Physician and Scientist Training Program in Urologic Research*:** NIDDK and the American Foundation for Urologic Diseases. Supports T32 training grants and K12 mentored clinical scientist development program awards (RFA-DK-98-005).

***R21 Fast Track Grants For Parkinson's Disease Research*:** NINDS, National Institute on Deafness and Other Communication Disorders, NIEHS, NIMH, the Michael J. Fox Foundation for Parkinson's Research, the Parkinson's Disease Foundation/National Parkinson's Foundation, and the Parkinson's Alliance. Supports R21 exploratory/developmental research grants (RFA-NS-02-006).

CENTERS FOR DISEASE CONTROL AND PREVENTION (CDC)

The CDC Foundation

www.cdcfoundation.org/

Established by Congress in 1992, the foundation forges partnerships with CDC to boost its programs. As an independent nonprofit organization, the foundation can accept funding and create programs that help donors and CDC scientists achieve common goals. It can find funding partners, negotiate deals, hire people, manage program budgets, identify experts, and report to donors. In the period 2002 to 2003, the foundation's revenues were $17.1 million and expenses were $10.2 million, of which $8.1 million were expended through cost-reimbursement agreements for programs. Thirty-seven corporations and 23 foundations that were supporting programs initiated as of July 2000 or are currently active are listed at the foundation website. Twenty-four global health programs with their partners were listed in July 2004, including:

- ***Asian Rotavirus Surveillance Program—Phase II*:** GlaxoSmithKline and Program for Appropriate Technology in Health
- ***Development of Rapid Assessment Methods and Tools for Displaced Persons*:** the Andrew W. Mellon Foundation

• ***Global Field Epidemiology and Laboratory Training Program—Kenya*:** Ellison Medical Foundation
• ***Lilly International Laboratory Fellowships*:** Eli Lilly and Company
• ***STD Control in the Russian Federation*:** Becton Dickinson and Company.

The Foundation also supports programs that promote healthy lifestyles, including:

• ***Avon-CDC Foundation Mobile Access Program*:** Avon Foundation
• ***Price Fellowships for HIV Prevention Leadership*:** Price Foundation
• ***Promoting Better Health for Young People through Physical Activity and Sports*:** MetLife Foundation

Among the research and education programs supported are:

• ***Antimicrobial Resistant Bacteria Educational Program*:** AB Biodisk, Abbott Laboratories, Becton Dickinson and Company, bioMérieux, Inc., Dade Microscan, Inc., Merck & Co., Inc., Ortho-McNeil Pharmaceutical, Inc., Roche, and GlaxoSmithKline
• ***Applied Epidemiology Training Program for Medical Students*:** Pfizer Inc.
• ***Estimation of Prevalence of Erectile Dysfunction in the U.S.*:** National Foundation for Sexual Health Medicine, Inc. and Pfizer Inc.

NATIONAL SCIENCE FOUNDATION (NSF)

Engineering Research Centers Program (ERC)

www.nsf.gov/pubs/2004/nsf04570/nsf04570.htm
www.eng.nsf.gov/eec/programs/index.htm#centers

NSF's ERC Program was created in 1985 to develop a government-industry-university partnership to strengthen the competitive position of U.S. firms in world trade. ERCs develop and maintain partnerships with member firms and other practitioner organizations. Member organizations serve on ERC's Industrial/Practitioner Advisory Board and are expected to provide access to key industrial facilities and personnel for ERC faculty and students, knowledge of industrial practice, and needs for future technological innovation. The research centers are funded by the National Science Foundation (80 percent) and by nonfederal cash and in-kind resources from industry, states, and other sources (20 percent). Members pay cash membership fees. Members also may provide the center in-kind and sponsored project support and/or provide support directly to ERC faculty for relevant sponsored projects. Some centers also receive cash and in-kind donations from nonmember organizations. Cost sharing at a level equal to 20 percent of the total amount requested from NSF is required and must be shown and justified in the proposal budget. Annual funding for centers ranges from $3.1 million to $19.4 million. NSF's contribution ranges from $1.0 million to $3.0 million per year, averaging $2.5 million per year.

Industry/University Cooperative Research Centers Program (I/UCRCs)

www.nsf.gov/pubs/2001/nsf01116/nsf01116.htm

Initiated in 1973, NSF's I/UCRCs program develops long-term partnerships among industry, academe, and government. These university-based centers start with a small investment from NSF, which is intended to seed partnered approaches to new or emerging research areas. Each center is established to conduct research of interest to both the industry and the university with which it is involved, with the provision that the industry must provide major support to the center at all times. Centers are expected to gradually become fully supported by university, industry, state, and/or other non-NSF sponsors. NSF supports I/UCRCs through a cooperative leveraging mechanism. In FY 2000, NSF contributed approximately $5.2 million, a relatively small amount compared with the $68 million contributed by other funding sources. In FY 2003, I/UCRC research resulted in approximately $75 million in R&D funding investments by member firms. The total industrial R&D investment attributable to I/UCRCs in FY 2003 was approximately $100 million. Each center is expected to maintain at least $300,000 of industrial support through membership fees, have at least six industrial members, and a plan to work toward self-sufficiency from NSF.

Materials Research Science and Engineering Centers Program (MRSECs)

www.mrsec.org/home/

MRSECs are interdisciplinary materials research and education centers. They are expected to have strong links to and actively collaborate with industry, national laboratories, other universities, and other sectors. Interdisciplinary materials research and education centers are funded by NSF (90 percent) and by nonfederal cash and in-kind resources from industry, states, and other sources (10 percent). Contributions can be from any nonfederal source, including nonfederal grants or contracts. However, contributions counted as cost sharing toward projects of another federal agency may not be counted toward meeting the specific cost sharing requirements of the NSF award. The 2004 program solicitation (www.nsf.gov/pubs/2004/nsf04580/nsf04580.pdf) indicates that awards range from $1 million to $5 million a year with an average of $1.9 million a year. Awards are made for an initial duration of up to six years, but the level of funding for the last two of those years is contingent upon the outcome of a thorough external review.

Nanoscale Science and Engineering Centers Program (NSECs)

www.nsf.gov/home/crssprgm/nano/start.htm
www.nsf.gov/pubs/2003/nsf03043/nsf03043.htm

NSECs are interdisciplinary research centers that address nanoscale science and engineering research problems too complex and multifaceted for individuals or small groups of researchers to tackle separately. Each NSEC must include partnerships with industry, government laboratories, and/or other users of research outcomes. NSECs receive NSF funding (90 percent) and nonfederal cash and in-kind resources from industry, states, and other sources (10 percent). Cost sharing at a level equal to 10 percent of the total amount requested from NSF is required and must be shown and justified in the proposal budget. In addition, contributions counted as cost sharing toward projects of another federal agency may not be counted toward meeting the cost-sharing requirement. The centers are funded by five-year cooperative agreements at between $1 million and $4 million a year, depending on the scope of the proposal, and they are eligible to compete for one five-year renewal.

Partnerships for Innovation (PFI)

www.nsf.gov/home/crssprgm/pfi/

The PFI program was established in 2000 as a result of a Congressional appropriation of $8.5 million to initiate a new innovation partnership effort. Partnerships must undertake one or a combination of research, technology transfer, and/or commercialization; workforce education and/or training; or establishing the infrastructure to enable innovation activities to take place. The program supports partnerships of colleges and universities with state and local governments and private sector organizations, including for-profit firms, nonprofit organizations, other academic institutions, entrepreneurs and venture capitalists, trade and professional associations, and federal laboratories. The lead organization must be a college or university (California Institute of Technology, Eastern Iowa Community College, University of Florida, and Tufts University are among the institutions with programs in 2004) and at a minimum there must be private sector partners. NSF offers two- and three-year grants for up to $600,000 in total costs. The cost-sharing requirement is 10 percent of the total amount requested from NSF. NSF funded 58 partnerships, 24 in the first round ($21 million) of awards, 12 in the second round ($7 million), and 23 more in 2002 and 2003.

Science and Technology Centers: Integrative Partnerships Program (STCs)

www.nsf.gov/od/oia/programs/stc/about.htm
www.nsf.gov/pubs/2003/nsf03550/nsf03550.htm

Launched in 1989, STCs are science, mathematics, and engineering research centers established to promote these areas of study, initiate efforts to improve the quality of education in these areas, and combine the relevant resources at universities with federal laboratories and private industry to enhance the transfer of knowledge among these different groups. The centers (25 initially; 11 in 2004) are expected to conduct world-class research in a variety of disciplines with partner institutions or organizations from other sectors that invest intellectual resources in and provide funding for the center. These partnerships include multi-institutional collaborations with other universities and colleges, national laboratories, research museums, private sector research laboratories, state and local government laboratories, and international collaborations. STCs receive NSF funding (70 percent) and nonfederal cash and nonfederal cash and in-kind resources from industry, states, and other sources (30 percent). Cost sharing at a level equal to 30 percent of the total amount requested from NSF is required. STC budgets may range from \$1.5 million to \$4.0 million per year for five years, and each center is eligible to compete for one five-year renewal. As of 1995, the original 25 centers had generated \$1.48 in nonfederal support for every dollar of NSF funding. NSF anticipates there will be another round of funding for the program in 2005.

NATIONAL INSTITUTE OF STANDARDS AND TECHNOLOGY

Advanced Technology Program (ATP)

www.atp.nist.gov/

A government-industry partnership formed in 1990, ATP provides cost-shared multi-year funding to individual companies and to industry-led joint ventures to encourage the development of challenging, high-risk, high-payoff technologies. ATP has strict cost-sharing rules. Joint ventures (two or more companies working together) must pay at least half the project costs; they can receive funds for research and development activities for up to five years with no funding limitation other than the announced availability of funds. Large *Fortune* 500 companies participating as a single firm must pay at least 60 percent of total project costs. Small and medium-sized companies working on single-firm projects are not required to provide cost sharing of direct costs but must pay a minimum of all indirect costs associated with the project. ATP does not fund product development, instead entering into cooperative agreements and playing a substantial role by providing technical assistance and monitoring the technical work, business progress, and expenditure of federal funds. Private industry bears the costs of product development, production, marketing, sales and distribution. Between 1990 and September 2003, 709 awards were made, with 1,433 participants; ATP provided \$2.114 billion, matched by \$1.987 billion from companies. For FY2004, a single company can receive up to a total of \$2 million for R&D activities for up to 3 years. The range of funding is \$434,176 to \$31,478,000; the average is \$2,971,402.

ENVIRONMENTAL PROTECTION AGENCY

Health Effects Institute (HEI)

www.healtheffects.org/

Chartered in 1980, HEI is an independent, nonprofit corporation that conducts research on the health effects of pollutants from motor vehicles and from other sources in the environment. It is supported jointly by the U.S. Environmental Protection Agency and 27 automobile companies, and has funded more than 170 studies and published more than 100 research reports and several special reports. In FY 2003, HEI declared total revenues and support in the amount of $6,151,066 and total scientific expense of $4,667,397.

FOUNDATIONS

Alliance for Cervical Cancer Prevention (ACCP)

www.alliance-cxca.org/

ACCP was established in 1999 by a Bill and Melinda Gates Foundation five-year, $50 million grant. Made up of five international organizations: International Agency for Research on Cancer, Pan American Health Organization, EngenderHealth, and JHPIEGO (affiliated with Johns Hopkins University) and the Program for Appropriate Technology in Health, the alliance has a shared goal of working to prevent cervical cancer in developing countries.

American Institute for Cancer Research (AICR)

www.aicr.org/research/matching.lasso

AICR'S grants program funds research projects with matching support from for-profit corporations. The program gives companies access to leading researchers in the field of diet, nutrition, and cancer, and use of AICR's NCI-approved peer review system. The program provides up to $75,000 per year (plus 10 percent for indirect costs) for renewable, two-year grants, providing companies with a cost-effective means to support high-quality research efforts. Matching funds may result from tax-deductible donations from collaborating corporations or individuals. AICR reserves the right to decline outside funds deemed inappropriate or that may result in a conflict of interest.

Global Alliance for TB Drug Development (TB Alliance)

www.tballiance.org/

Launched in 2000, TB Alliance is a public-private partnership and not-for-profit organization based on the premise of shared risks and incentive for partners whose mission is to diminish the spread of tuberculosis by developing new medicines. A number of organizations (e.g., American Society for Tuberculosis Education and Research, Bill and Melinda Gates Foundation, CDC, International Union Against Tuberculosis and Lung Disease, Lupin Laboratories,NIH) provide advice, guidance, and support for the alliance. While preference is given to joint ventures involving institutions in TB-endemic countries, stakeholders are selected based on research and development capabilities. The alliance establishes clear, predefined milestones, specific criteria and go/no-go decision points, and designs innovative agreements leveraging intellectual property rights to ensure the availability of novel technologies. The alliance periodically issues requests for proposals, which are evaluated and considered for investment by a scientific advisory committee.

The Charlotte Geyer Foundation

www.charlottegeyer.org/

The Charlotte Geyer Foundation awards provide one year's funding to exceptional proposals to give investigators the opportunity of advancing and improving projects to the point at which they are able to successfully compete for an R01 or other award. In practice, these are one-year awards of up to $100,000 to researchers whose proposals have been reviewed by NCI and were ranked within ten percentage points of the NCI pay line. More than 100 proposals have been funded since 1991; 17 proposals were funded in the year 2003. More than 85 percent of the funded proposals go on to receive NCI funding.

Kleberg Foundation

Rat Genome Sequencing Project

www.hgsc.bcm.tmc.edu/projects/rat/

In 2001, the Robert J., Jr. and Helen C. Kleberg Foundation in San Antonio, Texas, gave $4.2 million to the Baylor College of Medicine in conjunction with a joint award from NHLBI and National Human Genome Research Institute (NHGRI) of $37.7 million to sequence the DNA of laboratory rats within two years. Baylor's Human Genome Sequencing Center was the lead institution in a sequencing consortium that also includes Celera Genomics, Genome Therapeutics, The Institute for Genome Research, The University of Utah, Children's Hospital Oakland Research Institute, Medical College of Wisconsin, and University of British Columbia Genome Sciences Center. The Rat Genome Sequencing Consortium completed a rough draft of the sequence of the rat genome in November 2002. A more refined sequence and three-way comparison of the rat, mouse, and human genome were published in the April 1, 2004, issue of *Nature*. According to the president of Baylor, "Seed funding from private philanthropic institutions has proven vital to Baylor's ability to secure large NIH grants. The recent $4.2 million commitment from the Kleberg Foundation provides an excellent example of such leveraging. This private grant helped us obtain a $37.7 million public grant to support the rat genome sequencing project."

Bovine Genome Sequencing Project
www.hgsc.bcm.tmc.edu/projects/bovine/

The Kleberg Foundation subsequently gave Baylor $2 million toward the Bovine Genome Sequencing Project, which initially was to be a three-year public-private collaboration between Baylor, Texas A&M University, the National Institutes of Health, the State of Texas, and several corporations (www.bcm.tmc.edu/development/kleberg.htm). The eventual contributors to the collaboration when it was launched in December 2003 were NHGRI, $25 million; U.S. Department of Agriculture, $11 million; State of Texas, $10 million; Genome Canada, $5 million; Commonwealth Scientific and Industrial Research Organization of Australia, $1 million; and three New Zealand companies, Agritech Investments Ltd., Dairy Insight Inc., and AgResearch Ltd., $1 million each. The sequencing is being carried out at Baylor and Genome British Columbia.

Cystic Fibrosis Foundation Therapeutics, Inc. (CFFT)
www.cff.org

CFFT is the nonprofit drug discovery and development affiliate of the Cystic Fibrosis Foundation. Among other activities aimed at boosting the pipeline of drugs for cystic fibrosis, CFFT offers milestone-based matching awards up to $25 million for preclinical and clinical research to companies to develop promising potential drugs. More than two dozen of these alliances have been formed. Through Therapeutic Development Network[2] (TDN) funding, CFF has created partnerships with the private-sector research firms Chiron, Proteome, Copernicus, SciClone, and Inspire. The network also can function as a contract research organization for small companies that lack expertise, providing access to CFF-accredited care centers and patients. In 2003, CFFT spent $12.9 million on research grants, $22.4 million on TDN awards to 18 clinical research centers, and $2.7 million on clinical and research fellowship grants.

International Malaria Genome Sequencing Consortium
www.tigr.org/tdb/e2k1/pfa1/

This public-private consortium, the first multicenter international basic science collaboration in the malaria field, was formed in 1966 to sequence the genome of the human malaria parasite *Plasmodium falciparum*, clone 3D7. The

[2]The Therapeutic Development Network was established by CFF to conduct early-phase clinical studies with novel therapies for CF.

publication reporting this genome sequence appeared in the October 3, 2002, issue of *Nature* (pp. 498-511). The genome was sequenced by The Institute for Genomic Research and the Malaria Program of the Naval Medical Research Center (chromosomes 2, 10, 11, and 14); the Wellcome Trust Sanger Institute (chromosomes 1, 3-9, and 13); and the Stanford Genome Technology Center at Stanford University (chromosome 12). The PlasmoDB website (plasmodb.org) at the University of Pennsylvania also provides access genome data produced by the consortium. The approximately $29 million project was funded in the United States by the Burroughs Wellcome Fund ($7.7 million), NIAID ($3.4 million), and DOD ($5.3 million), and in the United Kingdom by the Wellcome Trust ($12.5 million).

The Kresge Foundation

www.kresge.org/

The Kresge Foundation provides grants to institutions on a conditional or challenge basis to build their capacity, help them broaden and deepen their bases of support from the private sector, and encourage volunteer involvement in the fund raising effort and beyond. Foundation assistance is directed toward the maintenance or expansion of institutions rather than for program or operating support. Initially, grants were made directly to institutions; by the early 1960s, however, the challenge concept had become a formal component of the foundation's policies. In 2001, the foundation awarded 164 grants totaling $111.5 million. An example is a $750,000 grant made to Baylor College of Medicine to construct a Biology of Inflammation Center. To meet the challenge grant and complete the project, Baylor had to raise approximately $7 million. The 2003 Annual report notes that, since its establishment, the Foundation has awarded 8,364 grants totaling $2.028 billion.

Medicines for Malaria Venture (MMV)

www.mmv.org

MMV was established in 1999 and is a nonprofit foundation that operates through public-private partnerships. Its goal is to bring public, private, and philanthropic sector partners together to fund and provide managerial and logistical support for the discovery and development of new medicines to treat and prevent malaria in disease-endemic countries. Funding and support has been received from a number of organizations, including the Bill and Melinda Gates Foundation, ExxonMobil Corporation, International Federation of Pharmaceutical Manufacturers Associations, World Bank, Wellcome Trust, and the World Health Organization. As of April 2004, MMV had 21 projects and plans to expand its portfolio, following the September 2003 announcement that the Gates Foundation would continue to support MMV with $40 million over the next five years.

The Whitaker Foundation

www.whitaker.org/

In 1992, the Whitaker Foundation and NSF jointly offered research grants to engineers, physical scientists, and health professionals to find ways of reducing the cost of health care without compromising its quality. This was accomplished through a series of competitive grant programs that supported research and education in biomedical engineering at academic institutions in the United States and Canada. In 1993, the foundation made 12 awards for a total investment of $6.5 million; NSF made a similar investment. In 1994, the foundation collaborated on a one-year program with NCRR; the foundation made 4 awards totaling $3.8 million and NCRR made 3 totaling $3.6 million. The foundation plans to spend all of its assets and close in 2006, and will not consider new applications. In its final round of research grants, 44 new awards totaling $10 million were made to 34 U.S. colleges and universities. In the final round of construction grants, awards totaled $24 million to six universities; these leveraged other grants and gifts totaling about $90 million. From the start of the program through 2003, 414 fellowships had been awarded, representing more than $53 million.

STATE AND LOCAL GOVERNMENT

California Breast Cancer Research Program (CBCRP)

www.cbcrp.org

CBCRP was established in 1993 and is administered by a small staff in the Office of the President of UC. CBCRP is funded from a portion of the state's two-cent tax on tobacco, voluntary tax check-offs on state personal income tax forms, and individual contributions. In 2003 California taxpayers donated $646,664 via their personal state income tax forms. The program funds researchers at California institutions. Since 1994 CBCRP has awarded nearly $150 million in 569 grants to 62 institutions in California. In 2004, the tenth funding cycle, the program made 43 awards totaling $14.6 million. They include 14 career development awards (10 postdoctoral fellowships, 4 dissertations), 14 collaborative grants, 7 larger-scale projects, and 10 high-risk/high-reward IDEA (Innovative Development and Exploratory Award) grants pursuing novel approaches to breast cancer issues (www.cbcrp.org/media/pr/061604.php).

The program has co-funded a few awards with the DOD Breast Cancer Research Program, but the philosophy of the program is to fill gaps *not* funded by other research programs in order to jump-start new areas of investigation and foster new collaborations. In fact, the program's legislative mandate is to "fund innovative and creative research, with a special emphasis on research that complements, rather than duplicates, the research funded by the federal government and other entities." For example, in the clinical area, with NCI funding large clinical trials, CBCRP gives priority to small preclinical or pilot studies of new approaches to therapy. Although CBCRP is small relative to NIH, foundation, and industry funding of breast cancer research, it explicitly tries to "influence this larger research system to go in new, creative directions" by funding high-risk ideas that, if successful, can obtain funding from other sources. The program's annual report cites specific instances of IDEA grants that later received support from NIH, the Komen Foundation, and industry (www.cbcrp.org/publications/reports/page_08.php).

California Institutes for Science and Innovation
www.ucop.edu/california-institutes/about/about.htm

The institutes were announced by the state of California in 2000 as a way to focus public and private resources and expertise on research areas considered key in sustaining California's economic growth and competitiveness in the global marketplace. Four research centers have been established by the state government and supported by the state, UC, and private industry:

- California Institute for Bioengineering, Biotechnology, and Quantitative Biomedical Research (QB3)
- California Nanosystems Institute (CNSI)
- California Institute for Telecommunications and Information Technology [CAL-(IT)^2]
- Center for Information Technology Research in the Interest of Society (CITRIS).

The institutes, located on UC campuses, are basic research centers concentrating on complex scientific challenges that demand multidisciplinary strategies and state-of-the-art equipment and facilities. They are also intended to foster university-industry collaborations in the research and training expected to produce the next generations of high-technology products and scientists.

The state is investing $100 million over five years in each institute, which must be matched by two dollars in non-state funding for every state dollar. At latest count, QB3, CNSI, CAL-(IT)^2, and CITRIS were collaborating with 16, 30+, 40+, and 20+ companies, which were also providing substantial resources to the centers (www.ucop.edu/california-institutes/partners/partners.htm). The centers are also leveraging federal dollars. In 2002, CAL-(IT)^2 received a grant for $4.3 million from NIH to train students at the interface of biology and computer science, and in 2003 it was awarded $12.5 million over five years by NSF to develop information sharing tools and organizational strategies for first responders to disasters, after providing the seed money to develop the project. CNSI received an NSF grant for $17.7 million over five years to establish a nanoscale science and engineering center. CITRIS is co-awardee with the University of

Southern California of a $5.5 million grant from NSF and the Department of Homeland Security to develop a large-scale cybersecurity testbed for the development of new defenses against computer worms and viruses.

Indiana 21st Century Science and Technology Fund

www.21fund.org/

In July 1999, Indiana established a 21st Century Research and Technology Fund with an appropriation of $50 million dollars to stimulate the process of diversifying the state's economy by developing and commercializing advanced technologies. Awards have been made in three broad categories: science and technology commercialization, centers of excellence, and entrepreneurial activities. In addition the fund provides cost-share on behalf of federal proposals submitted by Indiana-based entities. The fund emphasizes the creation of academic- and commercial-sector partnerships, with awards based on peer review, requiring excellence in the science or technological objective and a clear commercialization plan. Significant leverage from the partners involved in the projects is expected. Awards are made for periods of up to two years in amounts of up to $5 million, though the fund's board has indicated that awards above $2 million will be uncommon.

Kansas Technology Enterprise Corporation (KTEC)

www.ktec.com

KTEC is a state-chartered corporation established in 1987 to stimulate economic development in Kansas by fostering innovation and development of technology. Among other types of assistance to businesses in Kansas, it administers the Applied Research Matching Fund (ARMF) program to seed and early-stage investment capital for Kansas entrepreneurs, with investment made through either a royalty agreement or convertible debentures, and any financial returns reinvested in other projects. Funding may be made to companies working alone or in collaboration with universities, business incubators, or other companies. In 2003, for example, KTEC entered into 13 ARMF agreements, in which KTEC invested $1.1 million, matched by $2.2 million in matching funds. The Technology Commercialization Seed Fund (TCSF) invests in companies working alone or in collaboration with universities, business incubators, or other companies. Companies must match ARMF and TCSF investment with 150 percent of the amount of KTEC funding (60/40 split). KTEC seeks a return on its investment through either convertible debentures, equity, or in some cases, royalty investments. The Strategic Technology and Research (STAR) Fund assists researchers at Kansas Board of Regents' universities compete for federal and private grants by helping to provide matching funds. STAR provides 75 percent of the matching dollars required by a federal program; the remaining 25 percent must be provided by the university through waiver of indirect costs, direct financial support, or support from non-institutional cosponsors. In cases in which a state matching requirement is not explicit, such as partnership programs, applicants may request STAR Funds to enhance their chances for a federal award or for industry funding. In FY 2003, KTEC investments resulted in 34 company startups, 54 technologies, 53 patents, and $1.64 million in royalties.

South Carolina Technology Alliance

www.sctech.org/

The alliance was established to prepare a technology-capable workforce, create a business environment friendly to technology-intensive companies, invest to expand the base of rapidly growing companies and start-up business, and invest in world-class university research programs directly linked to South Carolina industry. Funding comes from local, state government, technology entrepreneurs, various grants, personal contribution and from services provided to stakeholders.

Legislation signed in 2004 (Act 187) commits a total $500 million for technology-based economic development. It comprises three major provisions. The South Carolina Life Sciences Act facilitates borrowing up to $250 million for university construction and improvement projects encouraging research and technology-based economic development. Multiple tax credits for recruitment and expansion of large life science facilities are provided; to receive them, more than $100 million must be invested in the new facility and it must create a minimum of 200 full-time, high-paying jobs. The state is also allowed to issue up to $250 million in general obligation bonds to pay for infrastructure improvements. The Venture Capital Investment Act of South Carolina created two funds within the Department of Commerce. One is the South Carolina Venture Capital Fund ($50 million total; up to $5 million equity, near-equity, and seed capital of up to $5 million or 15 percent of the committed capital of the South Carolina based investor, whichever is less). The other is the South Carolina Technology Innovation Fund (administration contracted to a separate nonprofit, small grants connected to the state's research universities). The South Carolina Research University Infrastructure Act increases the state's debt limit by half a percent to provide as much as $250 million for facility and infrastructure improvements at the state's three research universities (Clemson University, The Medical University of South Carolina, and the University of South Carolina-Columbia). Projects must advance economic development and creation of a knowledge-based economy.

State of Ohio's Third Frontier Project

www.ohio3rdfrontier.org/

A $1.1 billion initiative, this 10-year project was established in 2002 to expand Ohio's high-tech research capabilities and promote innovation and company formation to create high-paying jobs. Research is supported by funds from appropriations and a bond sale for matching grants to private firms and organizations for economic development projects. The project includes the Third Frontier Action Fund ($500 million over 10 years), a Biomedical Research and Technology Transfer Fund, and Wright Centers of Innovation, a capital improvement program for research facilities ($500 million over 10 years). One partnership created under the project is the Center for Stem Cell and Regenerative Medicine established in Cleveland by Case Western Reserve University in 2003. Its industry partners include Athersys, Viacell, Aastrom, StemCyte, Copernicus, VirxSys, and Cognate Therapeutics The Center was awarded $10.8 million to build the facility and another $8.6 million to finance research. It must raise 2 dollars for every state dollar awarded.

Translational Genomics Research Institute (TGen)

www.tgen.org/

TGen began in 2002 as an effort by the state of Arizona to create a biotechnology industry. It involves academic affiliation agreements with the three state universities in Arizona and collaborative relationships and related formal agreements with research and clinical organizations in Arizona and nationally (e.g., the Mayo Clinic, Banner Healthcare, and Virginia Piper Cancer Center at Scottsdale Healthcare). As TGen's work progresses from basic science to translational research to clinical applications, its agreements with medical research and healthcare delivery entities will cover collaborative research, clinical trials, and shared use of facilities. Arizona's state government has committed $30 million to this effort over 10 years. Other key contributors include universities and colleges pledged resources and faculty support, the Flinn Foundation ($10 million), the Virginia G. Piper Trust ($5 million), the Salt River Pima-Maricopa Indian Community ($5 million), the City of Phoenix (donation of land and construction of research facilities), health care providers (e.g., Banner Health Systems), local corporations, and private individuals.

University of California Industry-University Cooperative Research Program (IUCRP)

ucdiscoverygrant.org/welcome.asp

IUCRP was created in 1996 at UC Berkeley as a matching grant program to fund university-industry cooperative research projects in the area of biotechnology. It expanded to include electronics manufacturing and new materials, communications and networking, digital media, and information technology for the life sciences. The program provides grants for collaborative research partnerships with industry, in which companies provide matching funds and both parties share in the project's results. Initially, UC provided $3 million, which was quickly expanded to $8 million by a $5 million contribution from the State of California. Within three months, the program received applications with commitments totaling nearly $8 million in cash from California biotechnology firms. In 1998, the State of California increased its contribution to $12 million a year, while UC continued to provide $3 million. In 1998-1999, matching funds from industry and private contributions exceeded $15 million. In 1999-2000, and during the 2001-2003 fiscal years, combined funding was between $50 million and $55 million a year, more than half of it from industry. The program's UC Discovery Grant is jointly funded by the state, UC, and California R&D firms. To qualify, the projects must have committed matching support (at least $1 of private funding for every $1 of public funding) that represents new investment by California businesses. On average, each state dollar is matched by $1.57 from industry and 68 cents from UC. In addition, each industry dollar qualifies for California's 24 percent tax credit on investments in university research.

CANADA

Genome Canada (GC)

www.genomecanada.ca/home.asp?l=e

In 2000, GC was incorporated to support a national genomics research initiative by funding large-scale, peer-reviewed genomics projects whose scale and scope are such that they cannot be funded through existing mechanisms, national or international. The organization received $160 million (CAD) from the national government to establish five genome centers across Canada and fund genomic research and infrastructure projects on a 50-50 matching basis. Subsequently, GC received additional government funding. As of 2004, more than $379 million had been awarded for 78 research projects and research platforms, matched by $848 million in funds pledged by other partners. According to Louis Siminovitz, emeritus professor, University of Toronto, and a National Academyof Sciences member interviewed by Thomas Caskey and Michael McGeary on April 19, 2004, the matching required from each project has proven to be a difficult hurdle in many cases. Initially, GC required all matching to be from private sources, but this proved infeasible and eventually provincial government funds were allowed to be counted as matching. The provincial governments, however, have different capacities and willingness to provide matching funds. The start of some projects was delayed for months after they were approved while the matching funds were secured. Some otherwise meritorious projects could not be funded for lack of matching. Principal investigators reported spending large amounts of time lining up and then securing matching funds.

Ontario Research and Development Challenge Fund (ORDCF)

www.ontario-canada.com/ontcan/en/rts/cf/cf_intro.jsp

Created in 1997 by the Ontario government, ORDCF is an $800 million (CAD) program with a mandate to promote research excellence and partnerships between research institutions and business. It supports ground-breaking research in emerging fields such as genomics/proteomics and photonics, as well as in established sectors such as biomedical, agri-food, communications, information technology, and automotive. Funding is open to research institutions (including hospitals, universities, and colleges) on a competitive basis, for longer-term discovery research of interest to the private sector and shorter-term research with more immediate industrial applications. Under the terms of the program, the province contributes 40 percent, private sources 40 percent, and the research institutions 20 percent of the cost of each project. To date, the province has invested $453 million in 104 research projects. Private sector and research institution partners have invested an additional $1.2 billion, bringing the total value of Challenge Fund supported research projects to more than $1.6 billion.

Structural Genomics Consortium (SGC)

www.sgc.utoronto.ca/
www.sgc.ox.ac.uk/

SGC is a $95 million (CAD) effort launched in April 2003 by a public-private partnership. The objective is to develop the infrastructure and technologies necessary to determine 200 human protein structures per year and, within the first four years, determine the three-dimensional structure of more than 350 medically significant proteins and deposit them in a public database. The consortium consists of the Wellcome Trust, GlaxoSmithKline, and four Canadian research funding agencies: GC, Canadian Institutes of Health Research (CIHR), ORDCF, and Ontario Innovation Trust (OIT). The sites will be the University of Toronto and University of Oxford. The Wellcome Trust and GlaxoSmithKline initiated the project and are contributing £18 million and £3 million, respectively ($52 million CAD). GC and the Ontario government's Research and Development Challenge Fund are each contributing $15 million. OIT is contributing $7.2 million and CIHR $6 million.

UNITED KINGDOM

Joint Infrastructure Fund (JIF)

www.wellcome.ac.uk/en/1/biosfgjif.html

The £750 million JIF initiative was launched in 1998 by the UK Department of Trade and Industry's (DTI) Office of Science and Technology (OST), the

Higher Education Funding Council of England (HEFCE), and the Wellcome Trust. The purpose of JIF was to provide UK researchers with major equipment and new or renovated facilities needed to conduct cutting edge scientific research. DTI and the Wellcome Trust put in £300 million each and HEFCE contributed £150 million. Through five rounds of awards, 153 projects at 42 universities have been funded by the program. The applications were reviewed for scientific excellence by expert advisory boards of the appropriate research council or, in the case of biomedical and biological sciences, of the Wellcome Trust. The second level of review and final decisions were made by a Joint Executive Committee co-chaired by the Director General of Research Councils and the Director of the Wellcome Trust. The committee included representatives from the Wellcome Trust, the Research Councils and HEFCE, Scottish Higher Education Funding Council, Higher Education Funding Council for Wales, and Department of Higher Education & Further Education, Training and Employment, Northern Ireland.

Science Research Investment Fund (SRIF)

www.ost.gov.uk/research/funding/infrastructure.htm

JIF (see above) was succeeded in July 2000 by the new £1 billion SRIF sponsored by the same three organizations: OST, HEFCE, and the Wellcome Trust. The Wellcome Trust put in £225 million. The £675 million from the government was for university science infrastructure with the awards allocated according to research excellence and research income rankings. Most of the Wellcome Trust's funding (£150 million) was for biomedical science infrastructure projects drawn from the highest quality applications not funded by the government because of fiscal constraints; the remainder was for replacement or renovation of biomedical research buildings. The same peer review process used for JIF is being used for SRIF. Universities were expected to contribute 25 percent of the cost from non-SRIF sources. The government added another $1 billion for a second round of funding, in February 2003, for which the non-SRIF contribution was reduced to 10 percent.

B

Biographical Sketches of Committee Members

Joseph Pagano, M.D. (***Chair***) received his undergraduate degree from the University of Rochester with honors in English and his medical degree from Yale University in 1957. He has been a member of the faculty of the University of North Carolina, Chapel Hill, since 1965 and is Professor of Medicine and Microbiology and Immunology. He is a member of the Institute of Medicine and the American Association of Physicians. He is a past member of the Awards Assembly of the General Motors Cancer Research Foundation and past president and chairman of the Board of the Association of American Cancer Institutes. Dr. Pagano is past member of the Board of Directors of the Burroughs Wellcome Fund. He is a recipient of the North Carolina Award in Science and Chair of the North Carolina Advisory Committee on Cancer Coordination and Control. He is the Lineberger Professor of Cancer Research and Founder and Director Emeritus of the Lineberger Comprehensive Cancer Center at The University of North Carolina-Chapel Hill, School of Medicine.

Dr. Pagano is an expert on tumor viruses, specifically the Epstein-Barr Virus. His research focuses on molecular mechanisms of viral latency and oncogenesis and antiviral drugs. He is consultant to cancer centers in the United States and Canada, chair of the Scientific Advisory Board of Trimeris, Inc., member of the Scientific Advisory Board of AlphaVax, Inc., and advisor to the Franklin Street Partners.

Eric G. Campbell is an assistant professor at the Institute for Health Policy and the Department of Medicine at Massachusetts General Hospital and Harvard Medical School. His main research interests lie in understanding the effects of academic-industry relationships on the process and outcomes of biomedical research, the effects of local health care market competition on the activities and attitudes of medical school faculty, and the impact of data-sharing and withholding on academic science. In addition, he is researching the role of organizational culture in promoting patient safety. Dr. Campbell has published numerous articles in professional journals and has delivered numerous presentations at local, national, and international conferences on health care policy, medical education, and science policy.

C. Thomas Caskey is president and chief executive officer of Cogene Biotech Ventures, Ltd. In addition, he was recently elected president of the newly formed Texas Academy of Science, Engineering and Medicine. Dr. Caskey also served as senior vice president, human genetics and vaccines discovery, at Merck Research Laboratories, West Point, Pennsylvania, and president of the Merck Genome Research Institute. He serves as an adjunct professor at Baylor College of Medicine, Houston, Texas. Dr. Caskey earned his medical doctorate from Duke University, Durham, North Carolina. He has received numerous academic and industry-related honors. He is a member of the National Academy of Sciences and the Institute of Medicine. He is past president of American Society of Human Genetics and the Human Genome Organization. He served as chair, Advisory Panel on Forensic Uses of DNA Tests, Office of Technology Assessment, U.S. Congress, 1989-1990. He was a member of the Committee on DNA Technology in Forensic Science, National Research Council, National Academy of Sciences, 1989-1991.

Robert Cook-Deegan is director of the Center for Genome Ethics, Law, and Policy at Duke's Institute for Genome Sciences and Policy. He is also research professor in Public Policy Studies and the Department of Medicine. Until July 2002, he directed the Robert Wood Johnson Foundation Health Policy Fellowship program at the Institute of Medicine, National Academy of Sciences. He worked on mental health policy, tobacco control, cancer policy, biomedical research policy, and federal R&D budgeting for 11 years at the National Academies, following a stint at the National Center for Human Genome Research, National Institutes of Health, in its inaugural year. He previously worked at the Office of Technology Assessment, U.S. Congress, for six years, joining OTA as a Congressional Science and Engineering Fellow directly from a postdoctoral position in molecular biology at the University of Colorado. He graduated from the University of Colorado Medical School in 1979 and from Harvard College (chemistry) in 1975. He chairs the Royalty Fund Advisory Committee for the Alzheimer's Association and the external advisory board of a four-site project on genetic testing for Alzheimer's susceptibility. He is secretary and trustee of the Foundation for Genetic Medicine and former chair of Section X (Social Impacts of Science and Engineering) for the American Association for the Advancement of Science, where he is also a fellow. From 1996-2003, he was a seminar leader for the Stanford-in-Washington undergraduate program. Dr. Cook-Deegan was a member of the Board of Directors, Physicians for Human Rights, 1988-1996, with whom he participated in human rights missions to Turkey, Iraq, and Panama.

MaryAnn Feldman is Jeffery S. Skoll Chair in Technical Innovation and Entrepreneurship and professor of business economics at the Rotman School of Management, University of Toronto. Dr. Feldman held the position of policy director for Johns Hopkins Whiting School of Engineering and prior to that she was a research scientist at the Institute on Policy Studies at the University. Dr. Feldman is on the Advisory Panel for the U.S. National Science foundation's Program on Societal Dimensions of Engineering. Her research and teaching interests focus on the areas of innovation, the commercialization of research, and the factors that promote technological change and economic growth. A large part of Dr. Feldman's work concerns the geography of innovation—investigating the reasons why innovation clusters spatially and the mechanisms that support and sustain industrial clusters.

Mary Ann Guerra joined the Translational Genomics Research Institute (TGen) as its vice president of Research Operations in early 2004. Ms. Guerra has an extensive background in business management and research administration, experience that ranges from basic research to clinical trials execution. Prior to her work at TGen, Ms. Guerra was executive vice president of the Matthews Media Group, Inc. (MMG), overseeing Business Development, Therapeutic Practice Areas, Communications and Public Relations, Human Resource Management and the Client Services Division. At MMG, she helped reorganize the company to become a strategic health communications firm that is research-based and results-oriented. From 1994 to 2001, she was deputy director for Management at the National Cancer Institute, the federal government's lead agency for cancer research, where she oversaw a budget in excess of $4 billion and more than 5,000 people. Prior to that, she held several senior executive positions at the National Institutes of Health. Ms. Guerra holds a BA in Communications from The Ohio State University and an MBA in science, innovation and technology from George Washington University. She is an accomplished speaker who has received multiple professional awards.

Musa Mayer is known for her work in cancer patient advocacy. Since 2001, she has served as a patient consultant with the Food and Drug Administration's (FDA's) Cancer Drug Development Program and as a patient representative with the FDA's Oncologic Drugs Advisory Committee. Her responsibilities involve representing patient interests, experiences, and needs in working along with FDA staff in the planning and conduct of clinical trials with pharmaceutical companies. Ms. Mayer has also participated as a peer consumer reviewer for the Breast

Cancer Group in the preparation of new Cochrane Reviews. As a freelance journalist and author, Ms. Mayer has published three books on breast cancer including, most recently, *After Breast Cancer: Answers to the Questions You're Afraid to Ask.* She is the author of *Advanced Breast Cancer: A Guide to Living with Metastatic Disease,* the only book of its kind. Ms. Mayer also writes feature articles on breast cancer for magazines, newsletters, websites, and medical journals, and she has been featured as a speaker at many conferences. She is a 15-year breast cancer survivor.

Frank E. Samuel, Jr., has served as science and technology advisor to Ohio Governor Bob Taft since August 2000. In this role, Mr. Samuel advises the governor on science and technology issues as they relate to economic growth for the State of Ohio and focuses on aligning state science and technology programs with Governor Taft's Third Frontier Project. As the science and technology advisor, he also serves as chair of the Technology Action Board (TAB) and the Biomedical Research & Technology Transfer Commission (BRTTC). The Board and the Commission were established to provide state support for creating early stage capital, developing new technologies, enhancing jobs and business opportunities in the state and improving the health of Ohioans. In July 2003, Mr. Samuel was appointed a member of the Third Frontier Commission, the three-person governing board that oversees the state's Third Frontier Project.

Prior to assuming his state position, Mr. Samuel served as president of the Edison Biotechnology Center, Inc., in Columbus, Ohio; president of the Health Industry Manufacturers Association (HIMA) in Washington, D.C.; practiced law in Washington, D.C., specializing in regulatory, legislative and other governmental issues affecting healthcare technology and services; and served in a variety of positions in the U.S. Department of Health, Education and Welfare, including Deputy Assistant Secretary for Legislation (Health). He has been a member of the board of directors of a dozen biomedical and health insurance companies and organizations. He is a graduate of Hiram College and Harvard Law School.

Samuel Broder, Executive Vice President, Celera Genomics, Rockville, Maryland, was a committee member until May 25, 2004.

C

Workshop Agenda

IOM COMMITTEE ON ALTERNATIVE FUNDING STRATEGIES FOR DOD'S PEER REVIEWED MEDICAL RESEARCH PROGRAMS

April 26-27, 2004
Lecture Room, The National Academies
21st and C Streets, NW
Washington, D.C.

OPEN SESSION

Monday, April 26

9-10:30 AM Greetings and opening statements about the charge to the committee by:
Joseph Pagano, M.D., Committee Chair (9:00)

- **Patricia Modrow**, Ph.D., CDMRP Ovarian Cancer Research Program (9:15)
- **Leo Giambarresi**, Ph.D., CDMRP Prostate Cancer Research Program Manager
- **Richard Kenyon**, Ph.D., CDMRP Breast Cancer Research Program Manager

10:30 AM-12:15 PM PANEL 1: STAKEHOLDERS (Robert Cook-Deegan, Moderator)

- **Fran Visco**, President, National Breast Cancer Coalition
- **Rick Atkins**, M.D., President and CEO, National Prostate Cancer Coalition
- **Ann Kolker**, Executive Director, Ovarian Cancer National Alliance
- **Michael Coburn**, President and CEO, Tuberous Sclerosis Alliance
- **Brenda Duffy**, President, Neurofibromatosis, Inc.

1:15-3:00 PANEL 2: EXAMPLES OF PUBLIC PRIVATE RESEARCH FUNDING (Eric Campbell, Moderator)

- **Amy McGuire**, Executive Director, Foundation for the National Institutes of Health
- **Robert Goldstein**, M.D., Ph.D., Chief Scientific Officer, Juvenile Diabetes Research Foundation
- **Gayle E. Lester**, Ph.D., Program Director, Osteoarthritis Initiative Public-Private Initiative, NIAMS
- **Carole A. Heilman**, Ph.D., Director, Division of Microbiology and Infectious Diseases, NIAID
- **Robert O'Keefe**, Vice President, Health Effects Institute

3:00-3:15 Break

3:15-5:00 PANEL 3: PERSPECTIVES OF NONFEDERAL RESEARCH FUNDERS (Samuel Broder, Moderator)

- **Alan Kinniburgh**, Ph.D., Vice President, Medical & Scientific, Leukemia and Lymphoma Society
- **Robert C. Wells**, J.D., Vice President for Government Relations and Public Policy, Affymetrix, Inc.
- **Ray Takigiku**, Ph.D., Director of Core Technologies, Procter & Gamble Pharmaceuticals
- **Donald C. Harrison**, M.D., Senior Vice President and Provost for Health Affairs Emeritus, University of Cincinnati

5:00-5:30 **Open microphone for public statements**

Tuesday, April 27

8:30 AM **Maria Freire**, Ph.D., CEO, Global Alliance for TB Drug Development, on lessons learned from the TB Alliance experience about public-private partnerships in biomedical research (Dr. Freire was previously head of NIH's Office of Technology Transfer) (introduced by MaryAnn Guerra)

9:15-10:00 **Queta Bond**, Ph.D., President, Burroughs-Wellcome Fund, on the roles of philanthropy and the federal government in biomedical research (introduced by Joseph Pagano)

10:00-10:15 Break

10:15 AM-12:00 PM PANEL 4: PERSPECTIVES OF ACADEMIC RESEARCHERS AND RESEARCH ADMINISTRATORS (Thomas Caskey, Moderator)

- **Mina J. Bissell**, Ph.D., Distinguished Scientist/Life Sciences Division, Lawrence Berkeley National Laboratory
- **Chung Lee**, Ph.D., Professor of Urology, Cell and Molecular Biology and Director, Prostate Cancer Program, Robert H. Lurie Comprehensive Cancer Center, Northwestern University
- **Susan Ehringhaus**, J.D., Associate General Counsel, Regulatory Affairs, Division of Biomedical & Health Sciences Research, Association of American Medical Colleges (former Vice Chancellor and General Counsel, UNC at Chapel Hill)
- **Hank Gardner**, Dr.P.H., Associate Vice President for Research and Professor, Environmental & Radiological Health Sciences, Colorado State University

1:00-2:45 PANEL 5: STATE PERSPECTIVES ON PUBLIC-PRIVATE RESEARCH COLLABORATION (Frank Samuel, Jr., Moderator)

- **Dan Berglund**, President and CEO, State Science and Technology Institute
- **Frank E. Samuel, Jr.**, Science Advisor to the Governor of Ohio
- **Marion H. E. Kavanaugh-Lynch**, M.D., M.P.H., Director, California Breast Cancer Research Program
- **Phillip A. Singerman**, Ph.D., Executive Director, Maryland Technology Development Corporation
- **Leslie M. Alexandre**, Dr.P.H., President and Chief Executive Officer, North Carolina Biotechnology Center

2:45-3:15	**Robert D. Wells**, Ph.D., President, Federation of American Societies of Experimental Biology, and Director, Center for Genome Research, Institute of Biosciences and Technology, Texas A&M University System Health Science Center, on the role of public-private partnerships in biomedical research (introduced by Musa Mayer)
3:15-3:30	Break
3:30-4:15	**J. Leighton Read**, M.D., General Partner, Alloy Ventures, Palo Alto, CA, on the roles of public funding and venture capital in biomedical research and biotechnology (introduced by Thomas Caskey)
4:15-4:45	**Andrew A. Toole**, Ph.D., Assistant Professor, Department of Agriculture, Food and Resource Economics, Cook College, Rutgers University, on the economics of collaborative public-private research funding (introduced by Maryann Feldman)
4:45-5:00	Wrap-up
5:00	Adjourn

D

Leveraging Public Investments with Private Sector Partnerships: A Review of the Economics Literature

Andrew A. Toole and Anwar Naseem
Rutgers University

1. INTRODUCTION

The purpose of this report is to summarize the discussion and findings in the economics literature on collaborative efforts in research and development (R&D). A collaborative R&D arrangement, or equivalently an R&D partnership, unites multiple participants in a structured relationship to conduct research and development activities directed toward one or more objectives. The breadth of this definition presents an immediate problem. How does one organize the tremendous number and variety of collaborative arrangements that fit this definition into a conceptually meaningful structure? Since the answer to this question depends heavily on the analyst's purpose, it is not surprising that no uniform structure exists in the economics literature. Some of the conceptual structures found in the literature organize R&D partnerships by the number and identity of the participants, by the alternative legal structures governing the relationships among partners, by the type of research and development activities conducted or by the stated objectives of the partnership arrangement.

From the literature, we identified five institutional forms of public-private collaboration: (1) government supported industry consortia; (2) industry-university collaborations; (3) federal laboratory-industry collaborations; (4) government grant programs in support of technology development and commercialization; and (5) global partnerships in health and agriculture. While our focus on public-private collaborations encompasses a diverse set of institutional arrangements and participants, partnerships involving only private participants fall outside the scope of this report. Hagedoorn (2002) and Hagedoorn et al. (2000) are good entry points into the literature on inter-firm R&D partnerships.

To one extent or another, all the contributions to this literature touch on at least one of four main thematic areas. These are the: (1) motivations of the various parties for participating (objectives, expected benefits); (2) potential risks to the participants (conflicts of interest, comprising public trust, legal liability, loss of proprietary information, compromising the research and educational mission of universities); (3) characteristics of the institutional forms identified above (legal form, intellectual property [IP] rights, governance); and (4) evaluation of the outcomes or perceived success of the institutional forms.

Standing back and looking at the literature as a whole reveals considerable variation in the detail and depth of understanding across these areas. A large descriptive segment of the literature concentrates on the motivations and potential risks of public-private R&D collaboration. A number of studies provide general descriptions of the institutional forms but, overall, they provide very little detail about the specific structure of the relationships within any institutional form. Structural detail would define the role of each partner in various areas such as the decision making hierarchy, the ownership of IP, the funding, the performance of work, and the evaluation of the work. There are some case studies that provide insights into these structural aspects of collaboration. A much smaller group of quantitative studies tries to measure the outcomes or use some indicator of success. Again, these focus on evaluating the alternative institutional forms.

In each of the following two sections, we systematically discuss the findings in the literature related to the thematic areas. For each partnership participant, section 2 summarizes their motivations and risks. Section 3 presents information on the structure and outcomes for the five institutional arrangements identified above. Section 4 concludes the report with some reflections on the key messages that emerge from this diverse literature.

2. MOTIVATIONS AND RISKS

A main thrust in the literature is to understand the incentives that motivate participants to form public-private R&D partnerships. Public and private agents are quite different. National governments, intergovernmental agencies, universities, for-profit firms, foundations, and nongovernmental organizations (NGOs) all answer to different constituencies, operate under different norms of behavior, and frequently pursue different sets of objectives.[1] How is it possible that these disparate parties have sufficient incentives to form a collaborative relationship?

[1]Paul (2000) discusses the definition and origin of the NGO category. Although foundations are often included in this category, we mention them separately because advocacy is not central to their mission, whereas NGOs such as Greenpeace have a strong advocacy arm.

The answer, according to the literature, is that each party gets something they value out of the arrangement. This value accrues through a set of participant-specific benefits. Moreover, the benefits can be separate and distinct from the formal objectives of the collaborative agreement. The benefits that flow to firms and universities, for instance, are more strongly linked to their "membership" and the actual performance of the R&D. For governmental entities, foundations, and NGOs, the expected benefits that motivate participation are more closely linked to the achievement of formalized partnership objectives. In rest of this section, we summarize the expected benefits and potential risks to partnership participants identified in the literature.

Why Do Governmental Entities Become Involved in Public-Private R&D Partnerships?

At the broadest level, governments view R&D partnerships with private agents as a mechanism to leverage both their limited financial resources and, when appropriate, their unique research capabilities to achieve social objectives. Governmental entities include intergovernmental agencies, such as the United Nations, World Bank, and World Health Organization (WHO), national governments, and specific agencies within national governments. This is clearly a diverse set of governmental institutions. The literature, however, points to three main social objectives/expected benefits that motivate government involvement in public-private R&D partnerships. These are to: (1) increase industrial competitiveness, (2) foster economic growth by mitigating market failures in research and innovation markets, and (3) more effectively meet agency specific mission-oriented needs through cost and risk-sharing.

The push to increase industrial competitiveness in the United States began in the late 1970s as a response to falling market shares and profits in several key industries, especially automobiles, consumer electronics, and later, semiconductors (Brooks and Randazzese (1998).[2] Competitive pressure, particularly from the Japanese, provided the impetus for a series of new pieces of legislation aimed at stimulating collaborative R&D efforts between industry, government, and universities. For instance, the Bayh-Dole Act of 1980 and its amendments allow universities and other performers of federally sponsored research to patent and license their research results with greater ease. By clarifying IP rights, this legislation was intended to increase the flow of knowledge and technology into the private sector. Several other pieces of legislation passed during the 1980s and 1990s established Cooperative Research and Development Agreements

---

[2]Similar pressures in Europe led to the establishment of the pilot ESPRIT program to support cooperative R&D in 1981. This evolved into the present day European Framework Programs on R&D. See Hagadoorn et al. (2000) for a discussion of the policy environment in Europe and Japan.

(CRADAs), the Advanced Technology Program, the Small Business Innovation Research Program, and the Small Business Technology Transfer Program. While we do not discuss the historical development of these legislatively mandated programs, Link and Tassey (1989) and Branscomb and Keller (1998) provide good treatments.

A second reason for government involvement in R&D partnerships is to foster economic growth by mitigating market failure in research and innovation markets. Seminal contributions to the economics literature in the late 1950s and early 1960s by Nelson (1959) and Arrow (1962) provide the rationale for government support of R&D. They point out that private firms are likely to under-invest in R&D activities in which the return to society is significantly greater than the firm's own private return. This wedge between the social and private return to R&D is the result of research "spillovers" that prevent firms from capturing the full stream of benefits from their initial investment. Two forms of spillovers are identified in the literature: knowledge spillovers and consumer surplus spillovers (Branscomb and Florida, 1998). Knowledge spillovers are typically associated with basic scientific and basic technology research. Since the returns to this research are highly uncertain and long-term, firms are likely to under-invest and government can increase social welfare by supporting this type of research. Consumer surplus spillovers are associated with product and process development. In this case, profits to an innovator firm may not be sufficient to justify the required R&D investment; however, from a social perspective, the value of the new product or process exceeds its development cost. Governments may increase social welfare by supporting the development of such a product or process.

Public-private R&D collaboration also serves as mechanism to meet agency specific mission-oriented objectives through cost and risk-sharing. Because this is the most common rationale at the individual agency level, it encompasses the broadest array of mechanisms and objectives, including all five of the collaborative categories identified in the introduction. One important example of this type of cost sharing is the industry/university research center. These centers typically combine state, federal, and university funding of a dedicated research center affiliated with the university. In the late 1970s, the National Science Foundation (NSF) began its Industry/University Cooperative Research Centers (I/UCRC) Program as a means to leverage federal research funding with industry and university funding. The perceived success of this program led the establishment by NSF of the Engineering Research Centers (ERC) Program in 1984 and the Science and Technology Centers (STC) Program in 1987 (Brooks and Randazzese, 1998). Cost-sharing and matching requirements are also being used to supplement traditional cost-reimbursement grant mechanisms at NSF, National Institutes of Health (NIH), and other extramural funding agencies. In section 3, we summarize these and other mechanisms in more detail.

What Are the Risks to Governmental Entities Involved in Public-Private R&D Partnerships?

One of the fundamental risks that government entities face when entering into public-private partnerships is the "R&D contracting problem." Noll and Rogerson (1998) describe the contracting problem within the context of government-university research grants; however, the same problems plague research-based partnerships. Because research produces new ideas and improved capabilities and competencies, research output is extremely difficult to measure. As a consequence, R&D procurement contracts cannot be written based on measurable outputs. Incomplete contracting introduces risk, because there is no direct incentive for researchers to conduct high-quality research. This point is reiterated in work by Poyago-Theotoky et al. (2002) within the context of university-industry partnerships. They formulate the incentive problem within a principal-agent framework. The funding agency, which is typically a governmental entity, is the principal, while the research performers, either industry or university, are the agents. The problem is that agents pursue their own self-interest and their actions may not be consistent with the best interests of the principal.

There are additional risks to governmental entities that are mentioned, albeit briefly, in the literature. One concern relates to public opinion and trust relationships between governments and their citizenry. Particularly in the context of global partnerships for health and agriculture, some observers believe that private partners will take control of decision making and use public resources for their own gain. Thus, the integrity of the governmental agency comes into question. Moreover, conflicts of interest can emerge from a careless choice of a private partner. For instance, in one of the WHO's partnerships, it was charged that the appropriate standards for the management of hypertension were jeopardized because of the influence of one private partner that stood to gain from lower standards (Buse and Waxman, 2001). Mowery (1998) also highlights cultural differences as a risk to successful partnering. In his example, different methods of research management created conflicts in a CRADA agreement between a Department of Energy (DOE) laboratory and a private firm. Further, legal liability issues are an additional risk to governmental entities, particularly in R&D partnerships directed toward drug development. Pharmaceutical firms have dedicated legal departments and spend millions of dollars to defend against law suits related to adverse reactions and deaths from drug therapies. As participants in drug development partnerships, government entities expose themselves to similar legal liabilities.

Why Do For-Profit Firms Become Involved in Public-Private R&D Partnerships?

The literature identifies a large number of potential benefits that may accrue to for-profit firms from R&D collaboration. Almost all of the theoretical and empirical work in this area focuses on inter-firm R&D collaboration rather than collaboration with governments or universities. Nevertheless, it is reasonable to expect that these same benefits carry over to public-private R&D partnerships.

In a recent survey, Hagadoorn et al. (2000) put together a comprehensive list of theoretical benefits from research partnerships. They group contributions into three categories of the literature: transaction costs, strategic management, and industrial organization theory. For transaction cost theorists, R&D partnerships are a hybrid organization form that stands between arm's length market transactions for knowledge production and in-house knowledge production. They see the emergence of partnerships as an efficient response to problems with market contracts to produce technical knowledge and as a better alternative to building the necessary capabilities within the firm. By forming a partnership, firms are able to establish greater control over knowledge production relative to the market and reduce costs and risk relative to complete in-house knowledge production.

Five alternate perspectives are reviewed from the strategic management literature. First, from a competitive strategy perspective, R&D partnerships allow firms to respond quicker to changing market needs and introduce new technologies faster. Second, partnerships are motivated by strategic network advantages. These networks can increase research efficiency via scale and scope economies, create research synergies by exploiting different organizational competencies, and provide greater power to influence the decisions of rivals. Third, the resource-based view highlights the benefit to firms from increased access to complementary resources external to the firm. Fourth, R&D partnerships allow for greater organizational learning by increasing the effectiveness of knowledge transfer to the firm. Finally, this literature emphasizes a "strategic options" approach in which high levels of uncertainty in knowledge production can be reduced through incremental resource commitments. R&D partnerships allow firms to avoid pre-committing to the full cost of developing a new technology.

Industrial organization theory focuses on the potential market failure in research and innovation markets due to knowledge and consumer surplus spillovers. A standard result in this literature, mentioned above, is that private firms under-invest in R&D from a social welfare standpoint. Hagedoorn et al. (2000) divide this literature, which is heavily game theoretic and mathematical, into non-tournament and tournament models. Non-tournament models, which focus on the extent of innovation, find that cooperative R&D can mitigate problems with under-investment in R&D by reducing spillovers.

Tournament models focus on "races" between firms where the winner captures a monopolistic return. The results in this literature are mixed. R&D investment may or may not increase depending on whether firms undertake substitutive or complementary R&D.

Contributors to the empirical and policy literature identify a number of additional, and sometimes overlapping, benefits to for-profits firms from R&D partnerships. Based on data from inter-firm research cooperation in the video display terminal industry, Link and Zmud (1984) find that firms want to maintain and increase market share. Mowery (1998) suggests that firms desire access to research results in universities and public laboratories and coordinate with other firms to create a common technological "roadmap" to guide future R&D investment. Hagadoorn et al. (2000) point out that a number of studies emphasize access to complementary research results as well as access to key university personnel, federal laboratory scientists, and a pool of qualified students for recruitment. Drawing on the experience of one firm in a CRADA relationship with a DOE laboratory, Mowery notes that the laboratory offered "unique capabilities, facilities, and equipment that in many cases could not be duplicated elsewhere" (Mowery, 1998:42). Another study by the Government-University-Industry Research Roundtable (GUIRR) adds that the knowledge base of the firm's employees will be enhanced and expanded through partnerships (GUIRR, 1999). Feller and Roessner (1995) suggest that firms gain methods and tools and not specific products or research findings from their collaborations with ERCs. Finally, firms participating in public-private partnerships can improve their corporate image. This is especially true in the context of global health and agricultural partnerships.

What Are the Risks to For-Profit Firms Involved in Public-Private R&D Partnerships?

In contrast to the volume of work highlighting for-profit firm benefits and motivations for R&D partnerships, there is surprisingly little commentary on the risks to private firms. In a 1998 GUIRR workshop on barriers to collaboration with universities, Francis Via, who is the director of Contract Research for the chemical firm Akzo Nobel, provided the most comprehensive list we could find (GUIRR, 1999). At the top of his list is mistrust among partners. Developing mutual respect and avoiding opportunistic behavior is critical. Other risks he mentions include publication issues, IP, and timing. Firms are very concerned with the potential leakage of proprietary information and with keeping information confidential until sufficient lead-time is developed. IP rights can be a problem when new technologies are jointly developed. There are a number of issues regarding the costs of securing and protecting IP and in establishing agreeable licensing arrangements and royalty rates. Further, Mr. Via stresses differences in time horizons as a risk for firms. Generally, firms work on short-time horizons relative to universities (and probably federal laboratories), and the consequences of missed deadlines can be much greater for a firm than for a public partner.

Why Do Universities Become Involved in Public-Private R&D Partnerships?

There is general agreement in the literature that access to money and technical knowledge are the most important factors driving university involvement in public-private R&D partnerships (Brooks and Randazzese, 1998; Powell and Owen-Smith, 1998; Jankowski, 1999; Hall et al., 2000; Poyago-Theotoky et al., 2002). Jankowski states, "Not only does such an approach offer opportunities for alternative funding in an increasingly constricted budgeting environment, but such partnership provides an essential means for undertaking work that is becoming evermore complex and multidisciplinary" (Jankowski, 1999:61). Poyago-Theotoky et al. (2002) add that a university with strong ties to industry can leverage these ties to attract "star" scientists to their faculty. Furthermore, they suggest that universities are interested in building long-term relationships that lead to sponsored research, in-kind support, and donations from firms.

A secondary motivation for university R&D collaboration with industry is to enhance student education and job prospects. NSF's collaborative center programs, particularly the ERC Program, requires an "education program that integrates research results into curricula for precollege and college students and practitioners, and teams undergraduate and graduate students in research and education" (NSF, 2004). Moreover, Stephan (2001) points out that industry-university collaborative research provides a chance for industry and students to get a "pre-employment" look at each other. This serves as a kind of informal "internship" opportunity. Further, she suggests student will have the chance to learn about industry salary and working conditions. On the other hand, Feller et al. (2002) find that the number of firms actually hiring graduate students through ERCs was relatively small. Their interviewees explained that cutbacks in corporate employment and active recruitment by competitors were the primary reasons.

What Are the Risks to Universities Involved in Public-Private R&D Partnerships?

A variety of risks to universities from R&D collaboration with industry have been discussed in the literature. At the broadest level, many observers see increasing reliance on industry funding as a threat to the university's "open science" norms of behavior. "Open science" refers to the free expression, exchange, and dissemination of new ideas. Threats to the free exchange of ideas from industry collaboration include limitations on the disclosure of research findings in the form of database restrictions or confidentiality agreements, publication delays and decreased communication between faculty or faculty and students. Brooks and Randazzese (1998) point to anecdotal evidence in the *New York Times* and the *Wall Street Journal* as well as quantitative research by Blumenthal and colleagues to illustrate these threats. Francis Via, commenting from an industry perspective on publication delays, states, "Many times, any early publication can alert competitors to a new fertile area of research. . . . Delaying publication for review will provide an 18-month lead for the industry partner" (GUIRR, 1999:19).

In addition to restrictions on the free exchange of ideas, there are concerns about how private research partners are influencing faculty research topics and creating professional conflicts of interest (Cohen et al., 1998). Brooks and Randazzese (1998) and Poyago-Theotoky el at. (2002) cite several studies that find a positive correlation between industry support and the conduct of more applied research and fear that the former is causing the latter. Many observers believe that reallocating the university research portfolio away from basic research toward applied research would be undesirable. Brooks and Randazzese (1998) also cite a study of financial disclosure practices in scientific publications. It finds that more than 33 percent of the authors failed to disclose a direct financial interest in the publication's results. Further, Harman and Sherwell (2002) provide five interesting case studies illustrating a variety of faculty conflicts of interest. Some of these disagreements eventually involved university administrators in a tangle of legal and political issues.

Stephan considers the possible impacts of faculty ties with industry on students and curriculum. She cautions that such ties have the potential to "divert faculty away from students and curriculum" toward more profit-motivated activities such as securing research funds, patenting, consulting, or commercialization activities (Stephan, 2001:200). Using anecdotal evidence, Stephan points out that the trust relationship between a faculty member and student is jeopardized, sometimes leading to legal action. Moreover, increased secrecy in the laboratory appears to diminish peer learning effects as students are increasingly hesitant to discuss potentially valuable or proprietary information.

Why Do Foundations and NGOs Become Involved in Public-Private R&D Partnerships?

We could not locate any literature describing the motivations for foundations and NGOs to become involved in public-private R&D partnerships. Generally, these organizations are active in very specific areas that are dictated by endowment guidelines or specific charters. At the same time, they are typically very resource-constrained and limited in the organizational and financial contributions they can make to an R&D partnership. One type of potential benefit to these organizations occurs when a foundation uses or "piggybacks" on the peer review process of the federal agency as a project selection mechanism, which saves the foundation the expenses of the application and peer review processes.

What Are the Risks to Foundations and NGOs Involved in Public-Private R&D Partnerships?

We could not locate any literature describing the risks to foundations and NGOs from participation in public-private R&D partnerships. Based on the piggybacking arrangement described above, in which foundations rely on a federal agency's peer review process to identify projects to fund, they lose some control over the projects they fund. They run the risk of piggybacking on a flawed or biased project selection process.

3. INSTITUTIONAL FORMS AND EVALUATION

In this section we discuss each of the five institutional forms identified in the introduction. Generally, there is little detail in the literature on the collaborative structures employed within each category. Of course, for many of the federal programs, broad structure is provided by the enabling legislation and the administrative agencies implementing these programs. When available, the best information on structural characteristics is provided by case studies. With respect to outcomes, we summarize the existing empirical work in the literature that attempts to evaluate the success or performance in the five categories. However, there are relatively few such studies. Mowery notes, ". . . surprising little effort has been devoted to evaluation of any of the legislative or administrative initiatives . . . " (Mowery, 1998:39).

Government-Supported Industry Consortia

Because most industry consortia are typically industry funded, government-supported industry consortia are a fairly special form of public-private R&D partnership, at least in the United States.[3] Under a strict definition, industry consortia are groups of two of more firms in the same industry that are potential competitors (Aldrich and Sasaki, 1995). The best-known U.S. examples of government-supported consortia are the Semiconductor Manufacturing Technology Consortium (SEMATCH) and the Partnership for a New Generation of Vehicles. In Japan, the best known examples are the Very Large Scale Integration Research Project, the Fifth Generation Computer Project, and the Opto-electronics Integrated Circuits Project.[4] Regardless of national origin, government-sponsored consortia share three common elements: (1) they are intended to address a high priority national competitiveness issue; (2) they have well defined and specific objectives; and (3) they focus on "pre-competitive" or "generic" research.

In the United States, the legal framework that allows competitors to undertake cooperative R&D was established in the 1980s. The National Cooperative

[3]R&D consortia are a subcategory of research joint ventures (RJVs). RJVs refer to all research contracting arrangements between two or more parties. See Katz and Ordover (1990) or Hagedoorn et al. (2000) for a discussion of definitions.

[4]There are numerous other consortia examples. In Western Europe, for example, the European Union Framework Programs and its predecessor, the ESPRIT program (Caloghirou et al., 2001), and the Alvey program in the United Kingdom (Quintas and Guy, 1995).

Research Act of 1984 (NCRA) was intended to reduce the threat of antitrust action against legitimate research joint ventures. The act establishes a rule of reason approach for antitrust proceedings that balances the procompetitive and anticompetitive effects of the research joint venture. The act also protects firms from treble damages in private antitrust suits as long as the research joint venture is registered with the Department of Justice (Scott, 1989; Katz and Ordover, 1990; Mowery, 1998; Hagedoorn et al., 2000). NCRA was amended in 1993 to include cooperative ventures in production.

The academic literature on industry consortia is quite large, even when restricting attention to government-supported industry consortia. While it is not feasible to summarize this literature here, the studies are generally of two varieties: (1) case studies or comparative case studies (Katz and Ordover, 1990; Grindley et al., 1994; Roos et al., 1998; Sperling, 2001; Thornberry, 2002) and (2) quantitative studies based on survey results (Aldrich and Sasaki, 1995; Link et al., 1996; Sakakibara, 1997). Given the complexity and diversity of consortia arrangements, we simply summarize some of the lessons on consortia design and management provided by Grindley et al. (1994) for SEMATECH.

Grindley et al. (1994) provide a detailed discussion of SEMATECH's evolution and a comparative analysis with other high-technology consortia in Japan and Europe. They highlight three complex design and management challenges that all consortia must face; (1) how to define the research agenda and projects to undertake; (2) how to transfer research results to participants; and (3) how to allow sufficient flexibility to permit change as industry needs and circumstances evolve. In contrast to most European consortia, SEMATECH's centralized management structure and strong industry control allowed it to address these problems more efficiently. Moreover, they point out that the feasibility and eventual success of consortia-style collaboration in other industries will depend on the structure of the consortium, the political and economic expectations of the sponsors, and the alignment between the research activities of the consortium and the competitive problems in the industry.

Industry-University Collaborations

As mentioned in Section 2, the NSF introduced the industry-university cooperative research center (I/UCRC) model in the late 1970s. The center model was expanded by the NSF into the Engineering Research Centers (ERC) Program in 1984 and the Science and Technology Centers (STC) Program in 1987. According to the NSF, there are currently more than 50 active I/UCRCs, 11 active STCs, and a total of 41 ERCs have been established since 1984 (NSF, 2004). Moreover, non-NSF centers have grown rapidly through university based initiatives, sometime winning support from state governments through competitions (Adams et al., 2001).

While these centers are quite different in their specific technological focus, objectives, and size, the NSF-supported centers share three broad goals. First, they support generic and precompetitive research relevant to industry needs. Generic R&D has the potential for wide applicability to many different products and processes while precompetitive R&D permits the evaluation of commercial potential but stops short of developing a specific prototype. Second, NSF centers strive to improve education and strengthen the science and engineering workforce. Third, the centers try to promote and accelerate technology transfer from universities to industry.

A recent study by Adams et al. (2001) explores how I/UCRCs influence patenting by and the R&D expenditures of member firm laboratories. Using survey data collected from 202 industry R&D laboratories, the authors find that industrial laboratories that belong to an I/UCRC are over twice as large and more science-oriented than their non-member counterparts. Further, they find I/UCRC member laboratories receive 2 percent more patents, although this effect is not statistically significant. With respect to R&D expenditure, I/UCRC member laboratories spend 2 percent more on average. For both patenting and R&D expenditure, the effects were larger for NSF-supported centers. However, their results are subject to one important qualification. Larger and more productive industrial laboratories may seek membership in I/UCRCs. With their data, the authors are unable to rule out the possibility that their results driven by this alternative direction of causality.

Santoro and Gopalakrishnan (2001) used survey results from 189 firms that are members of I/UCRCs to investigate how various factors like trust, geographic proximity, communication and university IP policies affect technology transfer. Since collaboration involves some loss of control over proprietary resources, a greater degree of trust can facilitate technology transfer. Using an indicator for the extent of technology transfer activities at a center as their explained variable, the authors' regression results show that greater trust significantly increases technology transfer activities. Geographic proximity and more generous university IP policies are also found to significantly increase technology transfer. Their measure of communication effectiveness, on the other hand, was insignificant.

Feller et al. (2002) studied firms that participate in NSF-funded ERCs. Their primary interest is to investigate the benefits and barriers to technology transfer from ERC participation. In the mid-1990s, the authors collected survey results from 355 firms and conducted telephone interviews with 20 respondents. These firms were participants in one or more of the 18 ERCs active in this period. While many of the benefits they identify were mentioned in Section 2, their survey results provide a ranking of benefits. Firms rated the following benefits as very important or extremely important (the percentage of respondents is given in parentheses): (1) to acquire and access new ideas (80 percent); (2) to be associated with an ERC whose research was close to the company's research interests (73 percent); (3) to access research expertise at the ERC (65 percent); (4) to keep up-to-date with university research in the field (58 percent); and to gain access to specific ERC faculty (56 percent). Among these, the extent of alignment of research areas between the firm and ERC that was the most important factor determining the magnitude of benefits reported by the firms.

They identify a number of barriers to deriving benefits from ERC participation. These include company-specific factors and inter-organizational differences. Company strategies and priorities are quite fluid, leading to frequent changes in product lines and personnel. Often times, these changes reduce or eliminate the value from participation. Moreover, they identify several institutional differences between firms and ERCs that act as barriers. These include different value systems, time horizons, and research priorities. Overall, the authors interpret these barriers as a potential threat to the long-term viability of individual ERCs. They note, ". . . industrial support of cutting-edge academic research appears to be fragile and contingent upon the availability of complementary public sector support" (Feller et al., 2002:473). When NSF support ends, as is required by program design, the leveraging rationale used by firms to justify participation will end as well.

Federal Laboratory-Industry Collaborations

CRADAs are government-industry partnerships designed primarily to commercialize a technology in a federal laboratory. The traditional mechanism of technology transfer has been to simply publicize results of federally sponsored research. Patent licensing, direct research grants, and research consortia are other ways that public sector technology can be disseminated (Day-Rubenstien and Fuglie, 2000). However, in a CRADA, federal laboratories enter into a contractual arrangement with a private firm to develop a technology and are not required to reveal any proprietary information. Moreover, the private firm can be assigned the rights to any IP arising from the partnership, although the federal government maintains a non-exclusive right to license the IP (Ham and Mowery, 1998). CRADAs were instituted under the Federal Technology Transfer Act of 1986, and they have grown in number from about 34 in 1987 to more than 2,500 in the mid-1990s (Guston, 1998). CRADAs are credited for the development of important new technologies, such as the anti-cancer drug Taxol and the AIDS drug AZT.

Although CRADAs have been existence for more than a decade, they have not been subject to much rigorous economic analysis, in part due to a lack of data availability (Cohen and Noll, 1995; Stiglitz and Wallsten, 2000). As a consequence, most prior efforts use the case study approach to analyze CRADAs (Cohen and Noll, 1995; Day and Frisvold, 1993; Ham and Mowery, 1998). In this section we review how CRADAs have been implemented by three federal agencies and the emerging lessons as reported in the studies of Ham and Mowery (1998) for DOE, Guston (1998) for NIH, and Day-Rubenstein and Fuglie (1999, 2000) for the Department of Agriculture (USDA).

CRADAs at DOE

Ham and Mowery (1998) report on CRADAs between DOE's Lawrence Livermore National Laboratory (LLNL) and industry. They examine in particular five CRADAs at LLNL to identify the management factors that contributed to the success (or failure) of the CRADA and the benefits that were realized by the partners. The five cases were selected to reflect the diversity of CRADAs in terms of project size and duration, size of the participating firm, and the mix of product and process technology.

Several important findings emerge from the Ham and Mowery (1998) study. First, they find that private partners are motivated to participate in the CRADA largely to access the unique capabilities of LLNL such as large specialized facilities and equipment and the ability to put together multidisciplinary teams that focus on specific tasks. This suggests that accessing unique DOE technologies is not the primary motivation for firms to get involved with CRADAs. The firms interviewed stressed that the generic benefits they derived by participating were more important as it improves their long-term scientific and technical capabilities. Second, the authors suggest that CRADAs are most effective if they build on the historic missions and capabilities of the laboratory, rather on the projects that focus on civilian use technologies which are often be distant from the laboratory's main mission. Ham and Mowery (1998) are critical of the treasure chest view of technology development which assumes that federal laboratories possess unique technologies that need only be further developed and commercialized by private partners. Third, the authors find that CRADAs are not well suited for all projects. In particular, if the project is a co-development project, as was true in four of the five examples they studied, then gaining IP rights for the jointly developed results was not the central motivation of the private partners. Since negotiation over IP issues often delays the implementation of CRADAs, the authors suggest that partners seek other, simpler, mechanisms for collaboration when IP is not a central concern.

CRADAs at NIH

Guston's (1998) study of CRADAs at NIH discusses some of the mechanisms of project implementation at NIH as well as the emerging lessons of NIH's experience. As with CRADAs in other federal departments, both public and private partners perceive some mutual benefit from entering into a partnership. For the private firm, a partnership with NIH gives it access to novel gene therapy techniques developed by NIH scientists. Similarly, NIH researchers gain from their private partners access to "proprietary reagents or to commercial-scale facilities for the production of potential new drugs" (Guston, 1998:231).

The criteria for implementing CRADAs at the NIH appear to be more stringent and focused then those in other agencies. First, the CRADA must be related to the primary mission of NIH in biomedical research. Second, as Guston writes "any CRADA [at NIH] must be a highly focused research plan advancing a scientific purpose that could not be more appropriately achieved through any other mechanism" (Guston, 1998:231). The use of CRADAs to fund normal research activities—such as equipment purchase, support of research fellows, and tests for collaborators—is discouraged.

In 1996, NIH initiated a new type of CRADA—the material transfer agreement CRADA (MTA-CRADA). Under a MTA-CRADA, NIH researchers can acquire proprietary research tools from private partners, but the scope of the agreement is much broader than a simple material transfer agreement. MTA-CRADA allows collaborations that are primarily over materials without having to negotiate over IP rights that would be required in more interactive collaborations.

Guston identifies several areas of contention regarding CRADAs at NIH. The first issue is access to technologies. CRADAs are generally accessible on a first-come, first-serve basis and do not involve the complexities of procurement and competitive bidding. This informal CRADA selection process opens the door to political difficulties, because firms might question the fairness of process, particularly for high value technologies. As long as the supply of CRADAs is greater than the demand, this is unlikely to occur, but it is potentially problematic if the NIH technology involved is keenly desired by the private sector. A second problem is that some firms may view CRADAs unfavorably because they have the potential of creating competitors especially in mature product markets. Although the evidence for opposition by established firms to new technology created through CRADAs is lacking, Guston still suggests that aggressive marketing of new technology may backfire.

Lastly the issue of fair pricing and IP in the context of CRADA remains unclear. All CRADAs initially contained a fair pricing clause while allowing the licensee to obtain reasonable profits. The clause was eliminated in 1995, partly in response to the uneasiness expressed by private research partners. However, the government maintains nonexclusive rights to license CRADA inventions made by private sector partners "for research or other Government purposes." More explicitly,

> the government retains the right to require third party licensing "on terms that are reasonable under the circumstances," but only in "exceptional circumstances" where the government determines that health, safety, or regulatory needs require it; such determination is subject to administrative appeal and judicial review (Guston, 1998:237).

Guston further writes that this language on the government's right to license is too vague and broad and requires clarification.

CRADAs at USDA

Even though agriculture was not the main focus of technology transfer initiatives that led to creation of programs like CRADA, USDA has extensive experience in establishing partnerships as evidenced by the fact that its CRADA program has been operating longer and has more agreements per appropriated dollar than that of any other federal agency (Day-Rubenstien and Fuglie, 2000). CRADAs at USDA have resulted in the commercialization of biopesticides, vaccines for chickens, and a chemical that, when added to water, reduces soil erosion.

As with CRADAs generally, the USDA program requires that the partnership be consistent with the department's mission, there must be no conflicts of interest, and fairness must be demonstrated in the selection of partners. Scientists at USDA laboratories are generally the ones to initiate a CRADA if they feel that an innovation they have developed has market potential. Private firms can also approach USDA to setup CRADAs if they find a particular technology to be a promising candidate for commercialization (the Agricultural Research Service publicizes its research advances through a variety of channels [conferences, workshops, Federal Register, etc.] and also maintains a database that reports on research).

A criticism of CRADA—and partnerships in general—is that it diverts public research from its central research missions. To address this issue, Day-Rubenstein and Fuglie (2000) study the pattern of research allocation for CRADA partnerships and compare it with the priorities of public and private research activities. Employing USDA's research classification system, the authors estimate the amount of research resources allocated to five technology areas. Since the five technology areas are broadly representative of agricultural research and show sufficient variation in social and private benefits, the authors assume that a large share of private research will be devoted to those areas with a large private-good component, whereas the public sector will be more focused on areas with high social returns. This leads them to hypothesize that in partnership mechanisms such as CRADAs, the allocation of research resources will "reflect a middle ground between the priorities of each partner." They find support for their hypothesis because the public share of resources allocated in CRADAs is higher for technologies with relatively higher social returns. However, since the average contribution of private-sector participants is approximately two-thirds of the funding for CRADAs at USDA, the authors suggest that USDA may be underutilizing these partnerships for areas with low private incentives and over-utilizing them for R&D in areas where strong private incentives exist. However, the authors caution in over-interpreting the data, which are based primarily on CRADAs involving small companies.

Government Grant Programs in Support of Technology Development and Commercialization

To supplement traditional grant and contract mechanisms and to promote greater technology transfer and competitiveness, policy initiatives in the 1980s and 1990s created the Small Business Innovation Research Program (SBIR), the Small Business Technology Transfer Program (STTR), and the Advanced Technology Program (ATP).

The SBIR program was established in the Small Business Innovation Development Act of 1982. To be eligible for the program, 51 percent of a firm's ownership must be held by U.S. citizens and the firm must have fewer than 500 employees. The original legislation mandated all federal agencies with an extramural research budget greater than $100 million to set aside 1.25 percent from their budgets for this program. This budget percentage was phased in over a several-year period. After the reauthorization of the program in 1992, the set-aside was increased to 2.5 percent of each agency's extramural R&D budget. In the 2000 reauthorization, the set-aside remained at 2.5 percent.

The legislation established three phases to the SBIR program. All applicants must start with a Phase 1 proposal. The Phase 1 project is intended to test the feasibility of a new idea. The feasibility study lasts from 6 to 12 months and the Phase 1 awards can be up to $100,000. Given the preliminary nature of the projects funded in this phase, one would expect a high failure rate. If the results of the feasibility study are favorable, firms may apply for a Phase 2 grant to move their idea into product development. The Phase 2 award is up to $750,000 and lasts for a two-year period. Finally, there is a Phase 3 to the SBIR program. This is an unfunded phase in which the companies are expected to commercialize their product or process. There is no direct government involvement in this phase.

The objectives of the program outlined in the original 1982 legislation have remained intact over the two subsequent reauthorizations, with only minor changes in emphasis. The 1982 Act identified the following four objectives:

1. To simulate technological innovation
2. To use small business to meet federal research and development needs
3. To foster and encourage participation by minority and disadvantaged persons in technological innovation
4. To increase private sector commercialization of innovations derived from federal research and development.

Although the 1992 reauthorization kept these objectives; it increased the emphasis on commercialization. Archibald and Finifter (2003) explore the extent to which the SBIR program at the National Aeronautics and Space Administration's (NASA's) Langley Research Center responded to the new commercialization emphasis. Based on project survey data, they find that there was a shift to projects with greater commercial potential following the 1992 reauthorization.

The academic literature on the effects of the SBIR program is split. Studies using survey data collected from SBIR participants, either at the project or firm level, consistently find positive program effects across a variety of indicators such as sales, employment and patenting (Audretsch et al., 2002; Archibald and Finifter, 2003; Audretsch, 2003; NIH, 2003). For instance, a national survey sponsored by NIH finds that 39 percent of their SBIR winners have realized sales on their projects (NIH, 2003:3-33). In stark contrast, regression-based evaluations using data on both participant and non-participant firms, such as Lerner (1999) and Wallsten (2000), do not find significant sales or employment effects from participation in the SBIR program. Although the SBIR award indicator is never significant in Lerner's study, he does find the interaction between awards and regional venture capital investment to be significant. Wallsten's findings are more pessimistic. In addition to finding no effect on employment in his sample of publicly traded companies, he finds that SBIR awards simply displace a firm's own R&D spending dollar for dollar.

The STTR program was created by the Small Business Research and Development Enhancement Act in 1992. It is intended to complement the SBIR program and shares the same multiphase structure as SBIR. The most significant difference between the programs is that STTR requires U.S. small businesses to partner with a research institution—a university, federal laboratory or other non-profit research institution. The research partner receives at least 30 percent of the awarded funds. There are currently five U.S. agencies participating in this program: DOE, Department of Defense (DOD), Department of Health and Human Services, NSF, and NASA. Each agency must set aside 0.30 percent of its extramural research budget for the program. To date, there are no published economic studies evaluating the STTR program.

ATP was established by Congress under the authority of the Omnibus Trade and Competitiveness Act of 1988 and amended by the American Technology Preeminence Act of 1992. It is administered by the National Institute of Standards and Technology (NIST) of the Department of Commerce. The program is designed to increase the competitiveness of U.S. industry by accelerating the commercialization of new scientific and technological discoveries and facilitating the refinement of manufacturing technologies. The program supports collaborative research on generic and precompetitive R&D problems (Hill, 1998).

As the administering agency, NIST is responsible for designing "focused programs," reviewing proposals, and monitoring awards. NIST laboratories are not allowed to participate in the ATP program. ATP awards are given to single firms or industry-led joint ventures. Single-firm awards are generally granted only to U.S.-owned for-profit companies, although foreign-owned firms may receive awards if there is a clear U.S. interest which is evaluated using a strict set of guidelines. Industry-led joint ventures must include at least two for-profit firms that meet ATP qualifications under the single-firm guidelines and may include nonprofit organizations, independent research organizations, government laboratories, and universities. Universities and government laboratories may participate in ATP projects as subcontractors or as members of a joint venture; however, they cannot submit proposals on behalf of the joint venture (Department of Commerce, 2004).

The amount, duration, and cost-sharing requirements for ATP awards differ between single-firm awards and joint-venture awards. Awards to single firms may be up to $2 million over a three-year period while joint venture awards may last five years with no funding limitation. Cost sharing may be in the form of cash or in-kind contributions. For single-firm awards, small and medium size companies must absorb the indirect/overhead costs of the R&D while large companies must provide at least 60 percent of total project costs. For joint ventures, cost sharing must exceed 50 percent of the total project costs. All IP that results from the ATP-supported R&D belongs to the for-profit companies and cannot be assigned to government laboratories, universities, or other nonprofits. These institutions may share in the royalties through licensing arrangements (see www.atp.nist.gov).

Noting that only 15 percent of federally registered Research Joint Ventures involve a university partner, Hall et al. (2001) investigate the role of IP rights as a potential barrier to university participation. For 38 ATP projects, the authors supplement data from the ATP program with a survey instrument that asked participant firms if IP rights created and insurmountable barrier. The results show that about 32 percent of the projects examined faced insurmountable IP barriers. Coding this indicator as a dichotomous variable, they use a Probit model to identify those factors systematically related to the existence of IP barriers. The regression results suggest that IP barriers are greater when the there is a higher ATP funding share, when projects have a shorter duration, and when lead participants had previous experience with universities as research partners.

In another paper, Hall et al. (2000) use ATP program data and survey data for 192 ATP projects to investigate the role and consequences of university participation. Before using Order Probit models to analyze their data, the authors review the motivations for industrial firms and the motivations for universities to form R&D partnerships. They posit that for-profit firms seek access to complementary knowledge, eminent researchers, and the reputations of elite universities, while universities, on the other hand, are primarily motivated by financial gain. With this backdrop, the regression results reveal that ATP projects with a university partner have a lower probability of early termination and that the industry partners in these relationships find it more difficult to assimilate basic knowledge required for project completion. Moreover, they find that university partners are not associated with the generation of new applications of the project technologies. On a positive note, university partners, either as subcontractors or joint venture members, do not seem to introduce any unexpected research problems into the project.

Global Partnerships in Health and Agriculture

In this section we review some of the key studies pertaining to partnerships in other countries, particularly those that are designed to address the significant health and agricultural needs of developing countries. A review of international partnerships can be instructive in the design of domestic partnerships because (1) the institutional and policy environments of international partnerships are often very different from that in the United States and (2) such partnerships are often complex arrangements that involve several participants (governments, multilateral institutions, foundations, and large corporations), with each participant having different mandates and constituents. Examining the genesis of such partnerships and how they are structured, especially in aligning the disparate incentive structures of the participants, may provide some lessons for the U.S. case.

Partnerships in International Health

Public-private partnerships (PPPs) designed to address the research needs of developing country health are a recent phenomenon (Buse and Walt, 2000). Historically, health-related programs such as those that sought to eradicate certain diseases in a developing country were done under the auspice of the national government, often with the help of foreign donors, foundations, and international organizations. Those projects were designed primarily to improve public health by immunizing against a particular disease or educating the most vulnerable population about prevention methods. Few, if any, of these programs were research-oriented with a view of developing new products; rather, they sought to strengthen the health infrastructure and capacity of the country.

The private sector was never a significant player, because raising health awareness and delivering vaccines was regarded as a public good and appropriately the function of government health agencies. Moreover, because the purchasing power of consumers in developing countries is small, the potential market for health products in developing countries was, and remains, commercially unattractive. Private-sector firms, therefore, have generally invested little in research on tropical diseases. For example, of the 1,223 new chemical entities introduced globally in the period 1975-96, only 13 were specific to diseases in the tropics (Webber and Kremer, 2001). However, even though market realities have discouraged private firms from investing in research on tropical diseases, they have discovered, in the process of research on other diseases, several drugs to treat diseases prevalent in the developing world. Private firms also possess many of the important patents and tools needed to undertake pharmaceutical research on tropical disease, although they do not do so because they are constrained by institutional and market barriers. These include, but not limited to, a weak health infrastructure for drug delivery, inadequate IP protection, and weak markets. To encourage more private sector funding, a variety of pull and push incentives have been suggested (see Webber and Kremer, 2001, for a summary), but they have yet to be implemented.

The scientific and technological capacity of the private firms in developed countries has been strengthened considerably over the years, due in large part to greater technological opportunities and stronger patent rights, but the public research sector in developing countries has remained weak. Funding constraints, low scientific capacity, and problems in gaining access to the most productive research tools has meant that public-sector researchers in developing countries have been unable to provide indigenous solutions to infectious diseases in their countries. This has resulted in a widening disparity in health between rich and poor countries. It has been estimated that in 1990, 80 percent of the disparity in death and disability adjusted life years between rich and poor nations was due to communicable diseases that can be prevented and for which drug treatment exists, although in many cases the drugs would need to be improved to suit local conditions and cultural practices (Widdus, 2001).

It is against this backdrop that PPPs in international health have their origins. The purpose of a PPP is to bring together the public and private sectors in an effort to solve some of the most intractable diseases pressures, which otherwise may not be solved if each sector acted on its own. The private sector, even though it has the necessary resources, is unlikely to undertake R&D, because the private returns to such research are low. The public sector, on the other hand, is handicapped by too few resources, even though such R&D activities have high social returns and serve the public good. By suitably aligning the incentives of the two sectors and leveraging their capabilities, it is felt that resources can be mobilized to conduct the necessary research.

Partnerships are created with different needs and outcomes in mind. As such, there exists a diversity of arrangements, which vary with regard to participants, legal status, governance, management, and operational roles. Widdus (2001) provides six reasons why partnerships in international health have been formed: (1) to develop a new product; (2) distribute a donated or subsidized product to control a specific disease; (3) strengthen health services; (4) educate the public; (5) improve product quality or regulation; and (6) coordinate multifaceted efforts.

Most partnerships are primarily based on meeting the first three objectives. Examples of product development partnerships include the Medicines for Malaria Vaccine (MMV) and the International AIDS Vaccine Initiative (IAVI). Partnerships that are based on the product donation by corporation include the donations of albendzole, eflornithine, and leprosy multi-drug therapy among others. Some of these donation-based partnerships go beyond the donation aspect, and have involved activities to ensure effective distribution and use (Widdus, 2001). Notable among partnerships meant to strengthen the delivery of health services is the Gates Foundation-Merck-Botswana Comprehensive HIV/AIDS Partnership. Although it is beyond the scope of this paper to discuss the specifics of every partnership—the Initiative on Public-Private Partnerships for Health lists some 70 collaborative relationships (www.ippph.org)—we focus instead on three drug and vaccine development PPPs, specifically MMV, IAVI, and the Global Alliance for TB Drug Development (Global Alliance).

A unique feature of the three partnerships is that they pursue a business model that exploits the venture capital approach to investing (Wheeler and Berkley, 2001). The partners pool their resources and skills around specific projects in an effort to fund research projects that meet a certain socially desirable objective. The term "social venture capital" has been coined to reflect the nature of these partnerships, which primarily focus on high-risk upstream research that seeks to convert scientific basic research into actual drugs. Another important aspect of social venture capital is that it involves multiple nonprofit public and corporate partners to fund competitively the research needed to meet the desired objective. The three partnerships are also different in that they have established themselves as autonomous legal organizations, which gives them greater management and governance control over their research activities. Box D-1 summarizes the key objectives of the three organizations mentioned.

The organizations are rigorous in their evaluation of specific projects and proactively seek to register and license projects that involve for-profit partners. To decide on which projects to fund requires a thorough understanding of the target diseases, available protocols, and constraints (Wheeler and Berkley, 2001). As such, the partnerships have established extensive knowledge databases about each disease that allow for effective identification and prioritization of the projects deemed to be most vital and likely to succeed. As with any venture capital, the partnerships screen potential projects for feasibility and disburse funds to selected projects. The Global Alliance and MMV use competitive calls for project proposals to identify promising research areas, whereas in the IAVI case, staff members seek and develop projects based on information from scientific meetings and the published literature and on the advice of experts.

If drugs are developed, the three projects seek contractual arrangements with private firms to make products available at affordable prices while providing a positive return on the investment. Since partnerships expect that collaborating firms will manufacture and disseminate the final product providing incentives to the firm requires that firms be granted access to IP rights to the product. The contrasting approaches in dealing with IP and affordability in IAVI and MMV are instructive. In the case of IAVI, investments in small biotechnology companies have been made that account for a large share of the recipient firm's capital, on the assurance that the product will be affordable in low-income countries. IAVI allows the biotechnology firm to retain developmental rights as long as the products are made available to public-sector organizations in developing countries at a reasonable profit which has been set at cost plus no more than 10

BOX D-1
Examples and Objectives of "Social Venture Capital" in International Health

International AIDS Vaccine Initiative: To ensure the development of safe, effective, accessible, preventive HIV vaccines for use throughout the world

Partners/Donors include: Foundation Marcel Merieux, Francois-Xavier Bagnould Foundation, National AIDS Trust, AIDS Vaccine Advocacy Coalition, Albert B Sabin Vaccine Institute, World Bank, UNAIDS, Rockefeller Foundation, AP Sloan Foundation, Bill and Melinda Gates Foundation, Department for International Development (DFID), Glaxo Wellcome, Levi Strauss International.

Medicines for Malaria Venture: To discover, develop and commercialize antimalarial drugs at a rate of one new product every five years and at prices that are affordable to the most affected populations

Partners/Donors include: Association of British Pharmaceutical Industries, International Federation of Pharmaceutical Manufacturers Associations, Wellcome Trust, Rockefeller Foundation, WHO, World Bank, Global Forum for Health Research, DFID, and Swiss Development Corporation.

Global Alliance for TB Drug Development: To accelerate discovery and/or development of cost effective new tuberculosis (TB) drugs that will (1) shorten the duration of TB treatment or otherwise simplify it completion, (2) improve the treatment of latent TB infection, and (3) be effective against multi-drug-resistant TB strains.

Partners/Donors include: American Lung Association, American Society for Tuberculosis Education and Research, Association of the British Pharmaceutical Industry, Bill and Melinda Gates Foundation, Centers for Disease Control and Prevention, European Commission, Lupin Laboratories, Novartis India, Ltd, Rockefeller Foundation, DFID, US AID, World Bank, and WHO.

SOURCE: Wheeler and Berkley (2001), with authors' amendments.

percent. The biotechnology firm, however, retains rights to offer the product to developed county markets without any restrictions on price. If the firm fails to deliver the product at an affordable price to the public sector in developing countries, IAVI retains "march-in" rights, i.e., the right to transfer the technology to another manufacturer. Even if IAVI exercises its march-in rights, the biotechnology firm to which the IP is assigned is allowed to keep its assets and can continue to market the product elsewhere. MMV, on the other hand, has invested in drug-discovery projects done by large firms and where the investment represents only a small fraction of the R&D budget of the firm. Under these circumstances, the expectation of the firm is not greater equity but that it will enter into a product development agreement with MMV in which MMV will have downstream rights to the technology which it could license. And although the issue of affordability in MMV has not been specifically addressed, the organization retains the right to develop the product if the commercial partner withdraws or fails to meet its obligations.

If firms are to divert their scarce resource into funding neglected diseases, it is important that such research activities has value to a firm and provides it with access to knowledge, technology, competitive advantage, or markets that they would otherwise not gain. At the same time, the ability to provide the most access to intended beneficiaries in developing countries requires that prices be kept low. A social venture capital organization therefore leverages its investment by negotiating to keep profit margins low. To compensate for lower profits in developing country markets, firms can be given exclusive licenses to market products in developed countries without price restrictions. For example, an HIV vaccine could be sold to high-risk groups in industrialized countries as can a vaccine to tourists and the military. Lastly, firms may be willing to participate in such partnerships if there are nonfinancial benefits as well. For example, partnerships can signal that a firm is a good corporate citizen, and for some small firms, it can be a showcase of its expertise and ability to deliver products. The risk of failure to firms from participating in projects can also be minimized by seeking funds to an array of potential products, allowing large companies to choose the most promising ones.

Partnerships in International Agriculture

The gap between rich and poor countries in the production of knowledge also pervades the agricultural sector. This has resulted in the markedly lower productivity of agriculture in developing countries and has perpetuated poverty in many countries. Furthermore, the diet of many in the developing world does not contain sufficient micronutrients; for example, it is estimated that 250 million children are at risk of vitamin A deficiencies, which leads to learning disabilities and blindness (Rausser et al., 2000). With the advent of agricultural biotechnology, there is much hope that not only can the productivity of staple crops can be increased but also that expression of micronutrients like vitamin A could also be attained. As in the international health area, there is recognition that productivity-enhancing technologies will not be developed without the collaboration of public and private institutions.

This is because many of the key tools of biotechnology necessary for developing novel and productivity enhancing plant varieties are proprietary and in the hands of private firms. While there are several ways that public research institutes or local firms can obtain patented biotechnology genes and tools, partnerships are being increasingly used as a mechanism to transfer proprietary technology from the private to the public domain. In return, the private firm gains access to the public sector's germplasm, plant variety assessment infrastructure, and the capacity to undertake upstream research. This suggests that, despite the different underlying incentives facing the private and public research sectors, sufficient common ground exists for agents in the two sectors to partner and develop useful technologies.

For example, the Brazilian Agricultural Research Corporation (EMBRAPA) leveraged its soybean germplasm assets to develop a partnership with Monsanto through which it could obtain Roundup Ready genes and access to plan transformation technology. Together, EMBRAPA and Monsanto have produced a series of herbicide-resistant genetically modified soybeans that Monsanto will sell through its extensive dealer network. Under the terms of the partnership, EMBRAPA receives royalties from the sales, and also a portion of the sales will go back to fund research on sustainable soybean production. A similar type of collaborative arrangement exists in Egypt where the local public research institute and Pioneer-Hi Bred jointly developed a new transgenic *Bacillus thuringiensis* (Bt) strain. In the collaboration, the Egyptian public system gains access to the expertise needed to develop the local strain of Bt (the innovation) and to educate its staff. The private-sector partner pays the legal costs of patenting the invention and has access to the new Bt strain for use in markets outside in Egypt.

For countries that do not possess a strong scientific capacity, international research centers or IP consortia that partner with private firms may be the only way to access proprietary technology. Such arrangements are thought to significantly reduce transaction costs and risk associated with developing a technology. For example, the Golden Rice Humanitarian Board—a public-private collaboration which includes the International Rice Research Institute, European government laboratories and the Syngenta Corporation—was set up to unravel the overlapping IP claims needed to develop vitamin A-enriched rice (Golden rice) for the poor. By establishing good faith agreements on the use of private-sector IP by academic researchers, the Board significantly reduces transaction costs relative to the case if the public sector had tried to access the technology on its own. Recently, several new multi-country programs have been initiated to obtain access to technology for the poor. The African Agricultural Technology Foundation is a nonprofit corporation funded initially by Rockefeller Foundation. It will license and hold technology from the major biotechnology firms with a humanitarian use license and then provide the technology free to its scientists in poor countries. In addition, the Australian-based institute, CAMBIA, is making information about patented technology more readily available and is developing nonproprietary technologies for biotechnology researchers in poor countries. Another recent initiative is the IP-clearinghouse program in the United States, which has the goal of making IP from universities and government research institutes more readily available. This program seeks to design a toolbox of biotechnologies for public sector researchers in industrialized countries.

It is important to realize that while partnerships may be desirable in many instances, they are not costless. Indeed a survey of partnerships in agriculture

(Spielman and von Grebmer, 2004) finds that transactions costs of establishing a partnership to be "excessively high." These costs include the direct expenses of meeting legal requirements, such as writing up contracts and enforcing agreements, as well as indirect costs of adapting to different organizational cultures. Such costs can be substantial for public sector partners who often do not possess the legal expertise to negotiate contracts with the private sector. Spielman and von Grebmer (2004) also identify risks to partners who engage in joint collaborative efforts. For the private firm, who is usually the provider of a key technology, the risks include the potential misuse or controversial use of the technology by the partner, end users, or third parties, which could result in legal, financial, or reputational liability for the technology provider. For the public firm, there is risk to its reputation from associating with private firms and developing controversial technologies. Since public sector research organizations are supported by taxpayers, any association with a private firm that is perceived to benefit unduly the private firm may lead to unwelcome scrutiny. In minimizing these types of risks, private and public sector participants incur costs that may diminish the incentives to form a partnership.

Pray and Naseem (2003) identify several characteristics of successful public-private joint ventures in international agriculture. First, both public and private partners have had something to gain from these collaborations. The gains do not have to be financial, although financial gains may provide the strongest incentive. Second, governments had the political will and ability to negotiate with private firms; in many countries this can be very difficult because of ideology and mistrust of the private sector. Lastly, partnerships require a budgetary commitment from the public sector partners, which has been financed by foreign donors.

4. CONCLUDING REFLECTIONS

The economics literature on public-private R&D partnerships is extremely varied and, except for some case studies and legislative guidelines, provides little detail on the particular structures used to organize and carryout partnership arrangements. Nevertheless, this section provides a series of brief reflections on the literature and its relevance for the IOM Committee on Alternative Funding Strategies for DOD's Peer Reviewed Medical Research Programs.

(1) The focus and character of DOD's Congressionally Directed Medical Research Programs (CDMRP) are central to defining and organizing potential partnership arrangements. For instance, research projects on topics such as understanding cellular function in cancer propagation, developing a new breast cancer diagnostic method, or conducting a clinical drug trial for a therapeutic candidate must be separated for the purposes of partnership definition and design. First, the fact that each of these examples involves research in cancer immediately limits

the group of potential nonfederal partners. It is unlikely, for instance, that a firm focused on cardiovascular research will be in the potential partnership pool. Thus, the focus area of the research is directly related to the potential partnership pool. Second, the character of the research relates to the degree of "spillovers" and its proximity to the market. Cellular function research is much more basic in character than a clinical study of a potential drug therapy. Consequently, it has a higher degree of uncertainty about expected payoffs and is more distant from the market. As indicated in Section 2, spillovers and proximity to the market relate closely to the incentives for private partners, especially for-profit firms, to become involved in partnership arrangements.

(2) Generally, the role of government in public-private partnerships is usually "research passive," in the sense that they define mechanisms, review proposals, provide funds, manage the accounting side of research contracts, and sometimes monitor or assess outcomes. The obvious exception to this is the CRADA mechanism in which government laboratories are "research active" partners that engage in the conduct of research. because CDMRP is an extramural research program, the role of DOD for this program will be "research passive" and rules out the CRADA mechanism as a potential institutional form of collaboration.

(3) Consortia, industry-university centers, the SBIR/STTR programs, and the ATP program have a strong industry orientation and extensive industry participation in defining projects and methods. While CDMRP might design a collaborative mechanism based on one of these institutional forms, it seems inevitable that the current structure of vision setting and project selection will need to be changed to incorporate, to some degree, the interests of private partners. Depending on how the collaborative arrangement is structured, any number of risks might be introduced, including conflicts of interest, issues of public trust and program credibility, legal liability, and research reorientation away from high risk basic research toward more developmental and applied objectives.

(4) While Lerner (1999) referred to the SBIR program as "public venture capital," the social venture capital model that has emerged in the context of international partnerships for health offers another possibility for CDMRP. A key aspect seems to be the creation of a separate legal entity with a different governance structure that can funnel money into projects and programs. This IS similar to the Foundation of the National Institutes of Health (FNIH), which was founded by an act of Congress in 1996 as a nonprofit organization. As a separate institution, FNIH has greater flexibility to accept and direct funds than the NIH itself (Pfizer Journal, 2003).

REFERENCES

Adams JD, Chaing EP, Starkey K. 2001. "Industry-University Cooperative Research Centers." *Journal of Technology Transfer*, 26(1-2):73-86.

Aldrich HE, Sasaki T. 1995. "R&D Consortia in the United States and Japan." *Research Policy*, Vol. 24:301-316.

Archibald RB, Finifter DH. 2003. "Evaluating the NASA Small Business Innovation Research Program: Preliminary Evidence of a Trade-Off between Commercialization and Basic Research." *Research Policy*, 32:605-619.

Arrow K. 1962. "Economic Welfare and the Allocation of Resources for Invention." Pp. 609-625 in *The Rate and Direction of Inventive Activity*, Nelson RR, editor. Princeton, NJ: Princeton University Press.

Audretsch DB. 2003. "Standing on the Shoulders of Midgets: The U.S. Small Business Innovation Research Program (SBIR)." *Small Business Economics*, 20:129-135.

Audretsch DB, Link AN, Scott JT. 2002. "Public/Private Technology Partnerships: Evaluating SBIR-Supported Research." *Research Policy*, 31:145-158.

Branscomb LM, Florida R. 1998. "Challenges to Technology Policy in a Changing Economy." Pp. 3-39 in *Investing in Innovation*, Branscomb LM and Keller JH, editors. Cambridge, MA: MIT Press.

Branscomb LM, Keller JH. 1998. *Investing in Innovation*. Cambridge, MA: MIT Press.

Brooks H, Randazzese LP. 1998. "University-Industry Relations: The Next Four Years and Beyond." Pp. 361-399 in *Investing in Innovation*, Branscomb LM and Keller JH, editors. Cambridge, MA: MIT Press.

Buse K, Walt G. 2000. "Global Public-Private Partnerships: Part I—A New Development in Health?" *Bulletin of the World Health Organization*, 78:549-561.

Buse K, Waxman A. 2001. "Public-Private Health Partnerships: A Strategy for WHO." *Bulletin of the World Health Organization*, 79:748-754.

Caloghirou Y, Tsakanikas A, Vonortas NS. 2001. "University-Industry Cooperation in the Context of the European Framework Programmes." *Journal of Technology Transfer*, 26(1-2):153-161.

Cohen LR, Noll RG. 1995. "Feasibility of Effective Public-Private R&D Collaboration: The Case of Cooperative R&D Agreements." *International Journal of the Economics of Business*, 2:223-40.

Cohen WM, Florida R, Randazzese L, Walsh J. 1998. "Industry and the Academy: Uneasy Partners in the Cause of Technical Advance." Pp. 171-199 in *Challenges to Research Universities*, Noll RG, editor. Washington, DC: Brookings Institution Press.

Day K, Frisvold GB. 1993. "Medical Research and Genetics Resources Management: The Case of Taxol." *Contemporary Policy Issues*, 11:1-11.

Day-Rubenstien K, Fuglie KO. 1999. "Resource Allocation in Joint Public-Private Agricultural Research." *Journal of Agribusiness*, 17:23-134.

Day-Rubenstien K, Fuglie KO. 2000. "The CRADA Model for Public-Private Research and Technology Transfer in Agriculture." In *Public-Private Collaboration In Agricultural Research*, Fuglie KO and Schimmelpfennig DE, editors. Ames, IA: Iowa State University Press.

Department of Commerce. 2004. "ATP Proposal Preparation Kit." [On-line.] Available: www.atp.nist.gov/atp/kit-04/final-kit.pdf.

Feller I, Ailes CP, Roessner DJ. 2002. "Impacts of Research Universities on Technological Innovation In Industry: Evidence from Engineering Research Centers." *Research Policy*, 31:457-474.

Feller I, Roessner DJ. 1995. "What Does Industry Expect from University Partnerships?" *Issues in Science and Technology*, 11(1):80-84.

GUIRR (Government-University-Industry Research Roundtable). 1999. *Overcoming Barriers to Collaborative Research*. Washington, DC: National Academy Press.

Grindley P, Mowery DC, Silverman B. 1994. "SEMATECH and Collaborative Research: Lessons in the Design of High-Technology Consortia." *Journal of Policy Analysis and Management*, 13(4):723-758.

Guston DH. 1998. "Technology Transfer and the Use of CRADAs at the National Institutes of Health." Pp. 221-249 in *Investing in Innovation*, Branscomb LM and Keller JH, editors. Cambridge, MA: MIT Press.

Hagedoorn J. 2002. "Inter-firm R&D Partnerships: An Overview of Major Trends and Patterns since 1960." *Research Policy*, 31:477-492.

Hagedoorn J, Link AN, Vonortas NS. 2000. "Research Partnerships." *Research Policy*, 29:567-586.

Hall BH, Link AN, Scott JT. 2000. "Universities as Research Partners." NBER Working Paper 7643, March 2000.

Hall BH, Link AN, Scott JT. 2001. "Barriers Inhibiting Industry from Partnering with Universities: Evidence from the Advanced Technology Program." *Journal of Technology Transfer*, 26:87-98.

Ham RM, Mowery, DC. 1998. "Improving the Effectiveness of Public-Private R&D Collaboration: Case Studies at a U.S. Weapons Laboratory." *Research Policy*, 26:661-675.

Harman G, Sherwell V. 2002. "Risks in University-Industry Research Links and the Implications for University Management." *Journal of Higher Education*, 24(1):37-51.

Hill CT. 1998. "The Advanced Technology Program: Opportunities for Enhancement." Pp. 143-173 in *Investing in Innovation*, Branscomb LM and Keller JH, editors. Cambridge, MA: MIT Press.

Jankowski JE. 1999. "Trends in Academic Research Spending, Alliances, and Commercialization." *Journal of Technology Transfer*, 24(1):55-68.

Katz ML, Ordover JA. 1990. "R and D Cooperation and Competition." Pp. 137-203 in *Brookings Papers on Economic Activity, Microeconomics*. Washington, DC: Brookings Institution Press.

Lerner J. 1999. "The Government as Venture Capitalist: The Long-run Impact of the SBIR Program." *Journal of Business*, 72:285-318.

Link AN, Tassey G. 1989. *Cooperative Research and Development: The Industry-University-Government Relationship*. Boston, MA: Kluwer Academic Publishers.

Link AN, Zmud RW. 1984. "R&D Patterns in the Video Display Terminal Industry." *Journal of Product Innovation Management*, 2:106-115.

Link AN, Teece DJ, Finan WF. 1996. "Estimating the Benefits from Collaboration: The Case of SEMATECH." *Review of Industrial Organization*, 11:737-751.

Mowery DC. 1998. "Collaborative R&D: How Effective Is It?" *Issues in Science and Technology*, 15(1):37-44.

NIH (National Institutes of Health). 2003. "National Survey to Evaluate the NIH SBIR Program," Department of Health and Human Services, July 2003.

NSF (National Science Foundation). 2004. Various program solicitations, available at www.nsf.gov.

Nelson RR. 1959. "The Simple Economics of Basic Scientific Research." *Journal of Political Economy*, 67:297-306.

Noll RG, Rogerson WP. 1998. "The Economics of University Indirect Cost Reimbursement in Federal Research Grants." Pp. 105-146 in *Challenges to Research Universities*, Noll RG, editor. Washington, DC: Brookings Institution Press.

Paul JA. 2000. "NGOs and Global Policy-Making," United Nations, Global Policy Forum, available at www.globalpolicy.org/ngos/analysis/anal00.htm.

Pfizer Journal. 2003. *Public and Private Funding in the Quest for New Cures*. New York, NY: Impact Communications, Inc.

Powell WW, Owen-Smith J. 1998. "Universities and the Market for Intellectual Property in the Life Sciences." *Journal of Policy analysis and Management*, 17(2):253-277.

Poyago-Theotoky J, Beath J, and Siegel DS. 2002. "Universities and Fundamental Research: Reflections on the Growth of University-Industry Partnerships." *Oxford Review of Economic Policy*, 18(1):10-21.

Pray C, Naseem A. 2003. "Biotechnology R&D: Policy Options to Ensuring Access andBenefits for the Poor." Agricultural and Economics Development Analysis (ESA) Working Paper 03-08, Food and Agricultural Organization (FAO), Rome, Italy.

Quintas P, Guy K. 1995. "Collaborative, Pre-competitive R&D and the Firm." *Research Policy*. 24:325-348.

Rausser G, Simon L, Ameden H. 2000. "Public-Private Alliances in Biotechnology: Can They Narrow the Knowledge Gaps between Rich and Poor?" *Food Policy*, 25:499-513.

Roos D, Field F, Neely J. 1998. "Industry Consortia." Pp. 400-421 in *Investing in Innovation*, Branscomb LM and Keller JH, editors. Cambridge, MA: MIT Press.

Sakakibara M. 1997. "Evaluating Government-Sponsored R&D Consortia in Japan: Who Benefits and How?" *Research Policy*, 26:447-473.

Santoro MD, Gopalakrishnan S. 2001. "Relationship Dynamics between University Research Centers and Industrial Firms: Their Impact on Technology Transfer Activities." *Journal of Technology Transfer*, 26(1-2):163-171.

Scott JT. 1989. "Historical and Economic Perspectives of the National Cooperative Research Act." Pp. 65-84 in *Cooperative Research and Development: The Industry-University-Government Relationship,* Link AN and Tassey G, editors. Boston, MA: Kluwer Academic Publishers.

Sperling D. 2001. "Public-Private Technology R&D Partnerships: Lessons from the U.S. Partnership for a New Generation of Vehicles." *Transport Policy*, 8:247-256.

Spielman DJ, von Grebmer K. 2004. "Public-Private Partnerships in Agricultural Research: An Analysis of Challenges Facing Industry and the Consultative Group on International Agricultural Research." EPTD Discussion Paper No. 113. International Food Policy Research Institute, Washington, DC.

Stephan PE. 2001. "Educational Implications of University-Industry Technology Transfer." *Journal of Technology Transfer*, 26(3):199-205.

Stiglitz J, Wallsten, SJ. 2000. "Public-Private Technology Partnerships: Promises and Pitfalls." In *Public-Private Policy Partnerships*, Rosenau PV, editor. Cambridge, MA: MIT Press.

Thornberry JB. 2002. "Competition and Cooperation: A Comparative Analysis of SEMATECH and the VLSI Research Project." *Enterprise & Society*, 3:657-686.

Wallsten SJ. 2000. "The Effects of Government-Industry R&D Programs on Private R&D: The Case of the Small Business Innovation Research Program." *RAND Journal of Economics*, 31(1):82-100.

Webber D, Kremer M. 2001. "Perspectives on Stimulating Industrial Research and Development for Neglected Infectious Diseases." *Bulletin of the World Health Organization*, 79:735-741

Wheeler C., Berkley S. 2001. "Initial Lessons from Public-Private Partnerships in Drug and Vaccine Development." *Bulletin of the World Health Organization*, 79:728-734.

Widdus R. 2001. "Public-Private Partnerships for Health: Their Main Targets, Their Diversity, and Their Future Directions." *Bulletin of the World Health Organization*, 79:713-720.